T0173187

THE ACUPUNCTURE POINT FUNCTIONS CHARTS AND WORKBOOK

of related interest

The Acupuncture Points Functions Colouring Book
Rainy Hutchinson
Forewords by Richard Blackwell, and Angela Hicks and John Hicks
ISBN 978 1 84819 266 9
eISBN 978 0 85701 214 2

The Yellow Monkey Emperor's Classic of Chinese Medicine
Damo Mitchell and Spencer Hill
Artwork by Spencer Hill
ISBN 978 1 84819 286 7
eISBN 978 0 85701 233 3

The Living Needle
Modern Acupuncture Technique
Justin Phillips
ISBN 978 1 84819 381 9
eISBN 978 0 85701 339 2

The Acupuncture Point Functions Charts and Workbook

Erica Joy Siegel

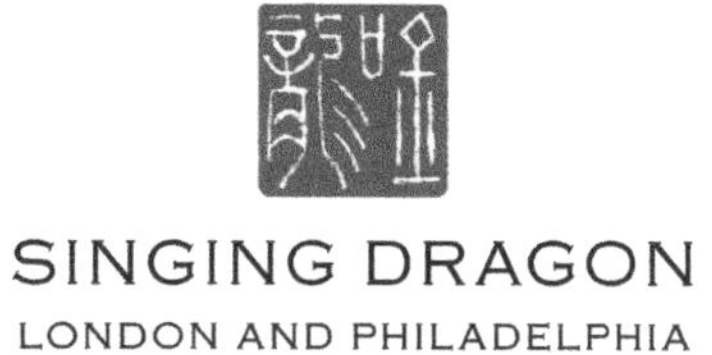

SINGING DRAGON
LONDON AND PHILADELPHIA

First published in 2019
by Singing Dragon
an imprint of Jessica Kingsley Publishers
73 Collier Street
London N1 9BE, UK
and
400 Market Street, Suite 400
Philadelphia, PA 19106, USA

www.singingdragon.com

Library of Congress Cataloging in Publication Data
A CIP catalog record for this book is available from the Library of Congress

British Library Cataloguing in Publication Data
A CIP catalogue record for this book is available from the British Library

ISBN 978 0 85701 390 3
eISBN 978 1 78775 009 8

Printed and bound in the UK

In Gratitude

I'd like to thank Peter Deadman and Giovanni Maciocia for their invaluable texts and dedication to Traditional Chinese Medicine, Darren Strecker for his help with modernizing and digitizing my chart illustrations, Mitch Harris for encouraging me to bring these charts to the world, and my family for their patience and love through the process.

Contents

The Acupuncture Point Functions Charts and Workbook is a visual study guide and quick clinical reference. Sources include Maciocia's and Deadman's 2015 revised acupuncture foundations books. It is a concise and architectural rendition. Each chart covers a meridian with its associated named acupuncture points and their functions. It covers the primary 12 meridians, the conception and governing vessels, and extra points. The extra points are on images of body areas along with cun measurements of all the primary acupuncture points.

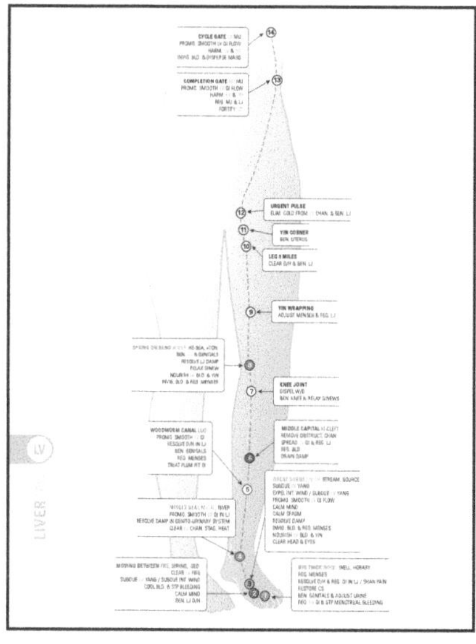

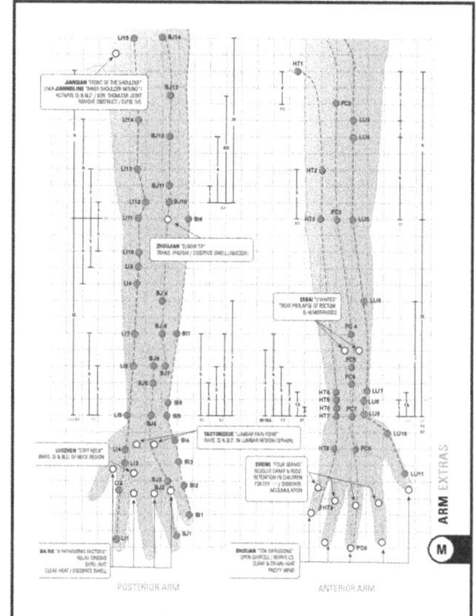

"Erica Siegel's acupuncture point diagrams were extremely helpful while learning point location and important functions. Her detailed drawings are not only accurate, but beautifully rendered – a welcome respite from textbooks."

– Elijah Hawken, M.S., L.Ac.

"I used Erica's point function charts during my TCM education. As a visual learner, I found them to be indispensable for all of my point classes, both in assisting me for exams and for imprinting in my mind the physical location of these points. The bold colors and clean, simple illustrations are still locked in my head after ten years of practice."

– Monica Kaderali, L.Ac.

"These charts are a MUST-have for every visual learner! Even after over a decade I can still see Erica's charts with point functions forever etched in my memory."

– Tracy Whynot, L.Ac.

"When I was studying in acupuncture graduate school we were constantly being tested on the location and function of points. Having a chart system that configured studying around two methods, meridians and body segments, was essential to my deeper learning of these pathways. These charts are clean to read, pretty to look at, and easy to carry around, which is an important function when trying to learn something deeply. Having something larger than a phone screen allows me to focus and learn without distractions."

– Mitchell Harris, L.Ac., Dipl.O.M., owner Eastern Integrative Health, Chair of Department of Clinical Procedure and Assistant Professor Pacific College of Oriental Medicine, Chicago

Introduction

While in graduate school at Pacific College of OM in San Diego, I had the opportunity to use ideas from past architectural education to create acupuncture point functions charts to assist myself in learning this plethora of information. As a visual learner, it was important to have the most efficient image memorization tools as possible. Having a whole channel or a large section of a channel with point functions right next to the points increased my cognitive ability to make the associations between the point locations and their functions.

The initial charts were hand drawn with pencil and marker. I did not publish or distribute them outside of my class. My colleague, Mitchell Harris, now a professor at PCOM, Chicago, suggested I revisit the charts and make them available to students and practitioners. Due to the 2015 revisions of Giovanni Maciocia's and Peter Deadman's major acupuncture texts it made sense that it was time to reinvent and edit the many changes in both texts of acupuncture point functions. Additional charts for measurements and extra point functions were created as well.

The charts are not only a learning tool but also a wonderful quick reference for practicing acupuncturists. To make the text in the charts as succinct as possible, there are many simple abbreviations, symbols, and color codes (see the next page for a key). Unless noted, all of the points are bilateral.

The second half of this book is a workbook. It is an opportunity to use creativity. There are empty spaces next to the acupuncture points to add notes, such as point indications, point depth, needle angle, and point combinations. Or use the spaces to test your knowledge of acupuncture point functions.

About the Author

Erica Joy Siegel is originally from New York. She attended Indiana University, Bloomington, and New York University's Gallatin School of Individualized Study. Her postgraduate work began with BTB Feng Shui training with GEO. She continued on to earn her Master's of Science in Traditional Oriental Medicine at Pacific College in San Diego, MSTOM. She is a nationally certified (NCCAOM) Acupuncture Physician practicing in Ponte Vedra Beach, Florida at Joy Vision Acupuncture, specializing in the treatment of ocular diseases. She formerly owned Indy Acupuncture & Health Services and Indy Downtown Community Acupuncture in Indianapolis, Indiana for 15 years. She served on the board of the Indiana Society of Acupuncture for ten years.

Abbreviations

TRIPLE JIAOS:

LJ: LOW JIAO
MJ: MIDDLE JIAO
UJ: UPPER JIAO

ABBREVIATED TERMS:

A.C.A.P.: ACTIVATE CHANNEL/ALLEVIATE PAIN
ALLEV: ALLEVIATE
BEN: BENEFIT
BLD: BLOOD
BRIGHT: BRIGHTEN
CHAN: CHANNEL
C.I.: CONTRAINDICATED
CREV: CREVICE
CS: CONSCIOUSNESS
D & D: DESCEND & DISPERSE
DISP: DISPERSE
ELIM: ELIMINATE
EXTING: EXTINGUISH
FULL CHEST: FULLNESS IN CHEST
FX: FUNCTION
GATHER: GATHERING
HARM: HARMONIZE
INVIG: INVIGORATE
LB: LOW BACK
MOD: MODERATE
N/V: NAUSEA & VOMIT
OBSTRUCT: OBSTRUCTION
PROMO: PROMOTE
PT: POINT
REG: REGULATE
REL: RELEASE
RESUS: RESUSCITATION
STAG: STAGNATION
STIM: STIMULATE
STP: STOP
SWELL: SWELLING
TRANS: TRANSFORM/TRANSFORMATION

SYMBOLS:

↓ DESCEND (ING)
↑ ASCEND (ING)
Ψ PSYCHO-EMOTIONAL
* SPECIAL FUNCTION

MERIDIANS:

LU: LUNG
LI: LARGE INTESTINE
ST: STOMACH
SP: SPLEEN
HT: HEART
SI: SMALL INTESTINE
BL: BLADDER
KD: KIDNEY
PC: PERICARDIUM
SJ: SAN JIAO
GB: GALL BLADDER
LV: LIVER
REN: CONCEPTION VESSEL
DU: GOVERNING VESSEL

POINT COLOR CODING:

WOOD
FIRE
EARTH
METAL
WATER
LUO
SOURCE
XI-CLEFT

8 PRINCIPLES:

EXT: EXTERNAL
INT: INTERNAL
-SED: SEDATION POINT
+TON: TONIFICATION POINT
TON: TONIFY
XU: DEFICIENT

EXTERNAL & BI PATTERNS:

D/C: DAMPCOLD
D/H: DAMPHEAT
W/C: WINDCOLD
W/D: WIND-DAMP
W/D/C: WIND-DAMPCOLD
W/H: WINDHEAT

Notes

Part 1

The Acupuncture Point Functions Charts

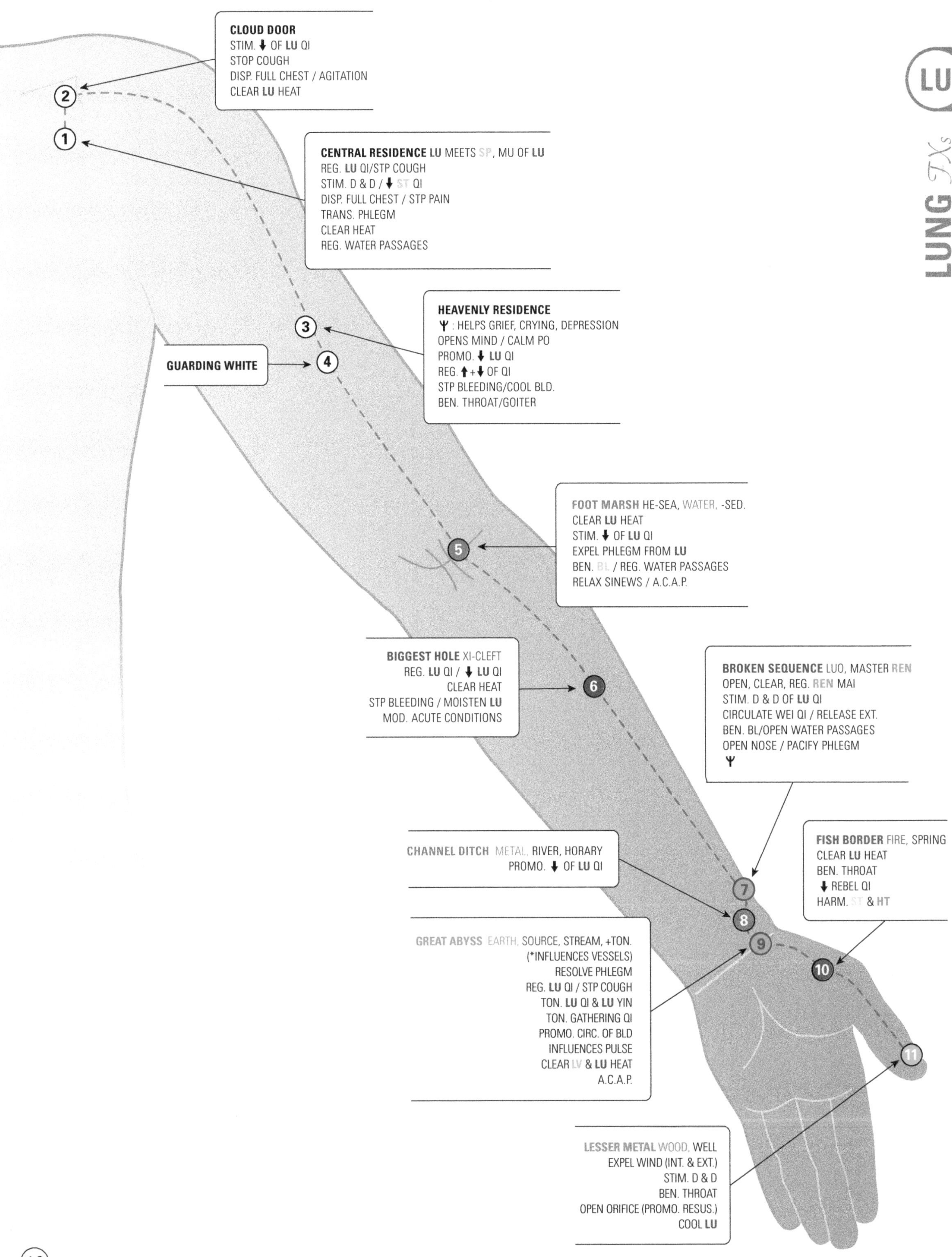

LU
LUNG FXs
CLOUD DOOR
STIM. ⬇ OF LU QI
STOP COUGH
DISP. FULL CHEST / AGITATION
CLEAR LU HEAT
CENTRAL RESIDENCE LU MEETS SP, MU OF LU
REG. LU QI/STP COUGH
STIM. D & D / ⬇ ST QI
DISP. FULL CHEST / STP PAIN
TRANS. PHLEGM
CLEAR HEAT
REG. WATER PASSAGES
HEAVENLY RESIDENCE
Ψ : HELPS GRIEF, CRYING, DEPRESSION
OPENS MIND / CALM PO
PROMO. ⬇ LU QI
REG. ⬆+⬇ OF QI
STP BLEEDING/COOL BLD.
BEN. THROAT/GOITER
GUARDING WHITE
FOOT MARSH HE-SEA, WATER, -SED.
CLEAR LU HEAT
STIM. ⬇ OF LU QI
EXPEL PHLEGM FROM LU
BEN. BL / REG. WATER PASSAGES
RELAX SINEWS / A.C.A.P.
BIGGEST HOLE XI-CLEFT
REG. LU QI / ⬇ LU QI
CLEAR HEAT
STP BLEEDING / MOISTEN LU
MOD. ACUTE CONDITIONS
BROKEN SEQUENCE LUO, MASTER REN
OPEN, CLEAR, REG. REN MAI
STIM. D & D OF LU QI
CIRCULATE WEI QI / RELEASE EXT.
BEN. BL/OPEN WATER PASSAGES
OPEN NOSE / PACIFY PHLEGM
Ψ
CHANNEL DITCH METAL, RIVER, HORARY
PROMO. ⬇ OF LU QI
FISH BORDER FIRE, SPRING
CLEAR LU HEAT
BEN. THROAT
⬇ REBEL QI
HARM. ST & HT
GREAT ABYSS EARTH, SOURCE, STREAM, +TON.
(*INFLUENCES VESSELS)
RESOLVE PHLEGM
REG. LU QI / STP COUGH
TON. LU QI & LU YIN
TON. GATHERING QI
PROMO. CIRC. OF BLD
INFLUENCES PULSE
CLEAR LV & LU HEAT
A.C.A.P.
LESSER METAL WOOD, WELL
EXPEL WIND (INT. & EXT.)
STIM. D & D
BEN. THROAT
OPEN ORIFICE (PROMO. RESUS.)
COOL LU
1
2
3
4
5
6
7
8
9
10
11

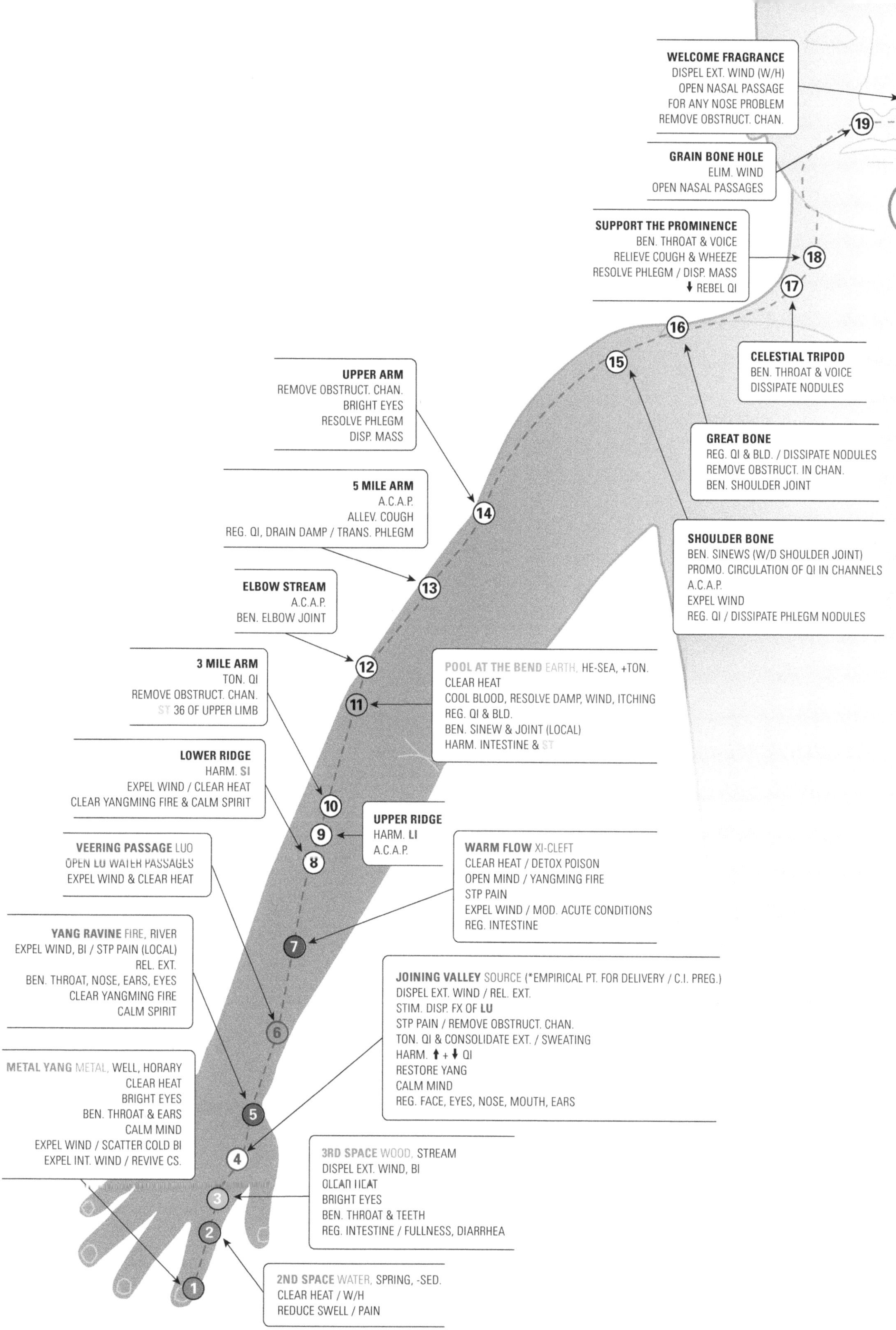

WELCOME FRAGRANCE
DISPEL EXT. WIND (W/H)
OPEN NASAL PASSAGE
FOR ANY NOSE PROBLEM
REMOVE OBSTRUCT. CHAN.
20

GRAIN BONE HOLE
ELIM. WIND
OPEN NASAL PASSAGES
19

SUPPORT THE PROMINENCE
BEN. THROAT & VOICE
RELIEVE COUGH & WHEEZE
RESOLVE PHLEGM / DISP. MASS
⬇ REBEL QI
18

CELESTIAL TRIPOD
BEN. THROAT & VOICE
DISSIPATE NODULES
17

GREAT BONE
REG. QI & BLD. / DISSIPATE NODULES
REMOVE OBSTRUCT. IN CHAN.
BEN. SHOULDER JOINT
16

SHOULDER BONE
BEN. SINEWS (W/D SHOULDER JOINT)
PROMO. CIRCULATION OF QI IN CHANNELS
A.C.A.P.
EXPEL WIND
REG. QI / DISSIPATE PHLEGM NODULES
15

UPPER ARM
REMOVE OBSTRUCT. CHAN.
BRIGHT EYES
RESOLVE PHLEGM
DISP. MASS
14

5 MILE ARM
A.C.A.P.
ALLEV. COUGH
REG. QI, DRAIN DAMP / TRANS. PHLEGM
13

ELBOW STREAM
A.C.A.P.
BEN. ELBOW JOINT
12

POOL AT THE BEND EARTH, HE-SEA, +TON.
CLEAR HEAT
COOL BLOOD, RESOLVE DAMP, WIND, ITCHING
REG. QI & BLD.
BEN. SINEW & JOINT (LOCAL)
HARM. INTESTINE & ST
11

3 MILE ARM
TON. QI
REMOVE OBSTRUCT. CHAN.
ST 36 OF UPPER LIMB
10

UPPER RIDGE
HARM. **LI**
A.C.A.P.
9

LOWER RIDGE
HARM. **SI**
EXPEL WIND / CLEAR HEAT
CLEAR YANGMING FIRE & CALM SPIRIT
8

WARM FLOW XI-CLEFT
CLEAR HEAT / DETOX POISON
OPEN MIND / YANGMING FIRE
STP PAIN
EXPEL WIND / MOD. ACUTE CONDITIONS
REG. INTESTINE
7

VEERING PASSAGE LUO
OPEN **LU** WATER PASSAGES
EXPEL WIND & CLEAR HEAT
6

YANG RAVINE FIRE, RIVER
EXPEL WIND, BI / STP PAIN (LOCAL)
REL. EXT.
BEN. THROAT, NOSE, EARS, EYES
CLEAR YANGMING FIRE
CALM SPIRIT
5

JOINING VALLEY SOURCE (*EMPIRICAL PT. FOR DELIVERY / C.I. PREG.)
DISPEL EXT. WIND / REL. EXT.
STIM. DISP. FX OF **LU**
STP PAIN / REMOVE OBSTRUCT. CHAN.
TON. QI & CONSOLIDATE EXT. / SWEATING
HARM. ⬆ + ⬇ QI
RESTORE YANG
CALM MIND
REG. FACE, EYES, NOSE, MOUTH, EARS
4

3RD SPACE WOOD, STREAM
DISPEL EXT. WIND, BI
CLEAR HEAT
BRIGHT EYES
BEN. THROAT & TEETH
REG. INTESTINE / FULLNESS, DIARRHEA
3

2ND SPACE WATER, SPRING, -SED.
CLEAR HEAT / W/H
REDUCE SWELL / PAIN
2

METAL YANG METAL, WELL, HORARY
CLEAR HEAT
BRIGHT EYES
BEN. THROAT & EARS
CALM MIND
EXPEL WIND / SCATTER COLD BI
EXPEL INT. WIND / REVIVE CS.
1

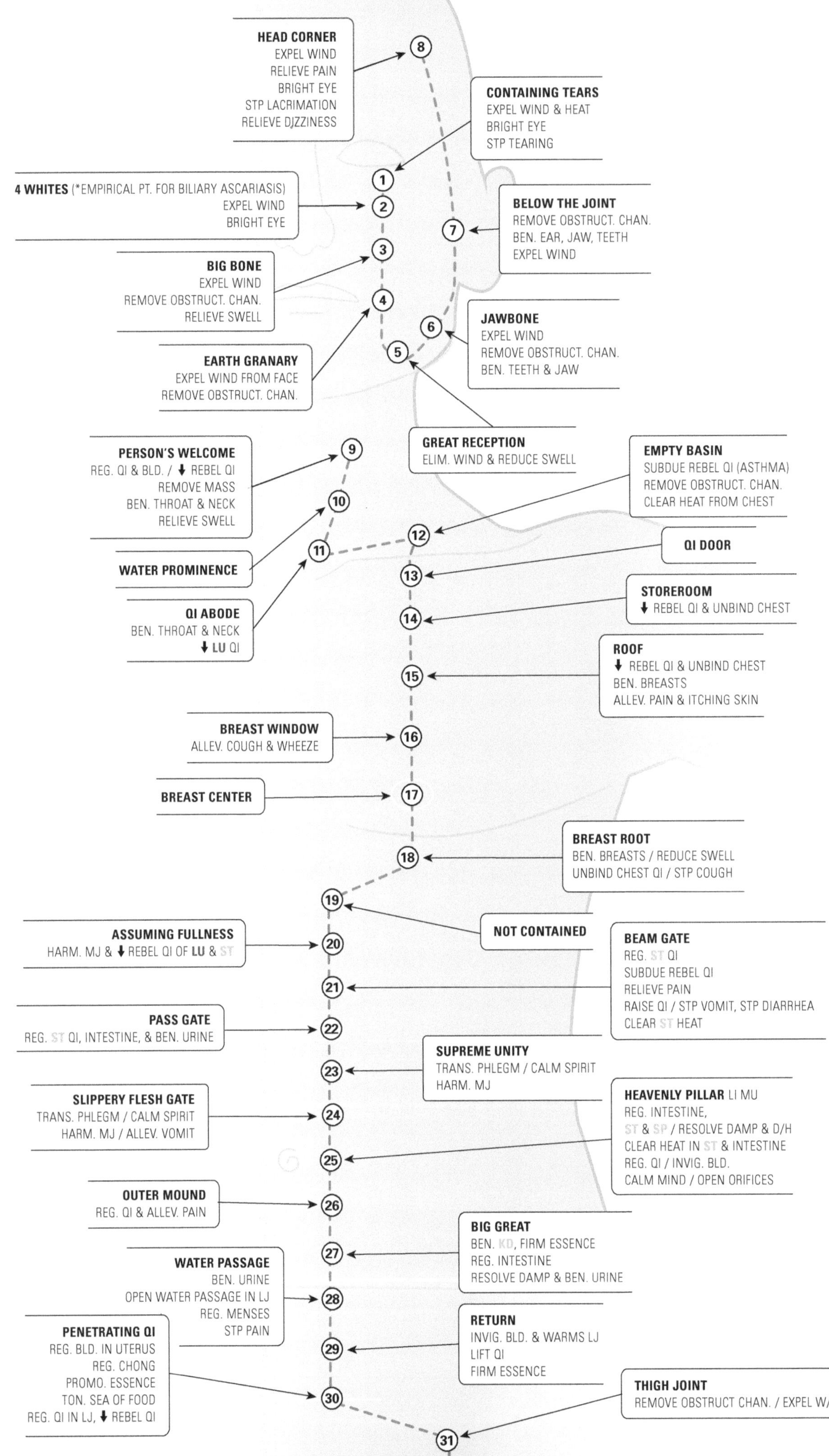

ST

STOMACH FX's

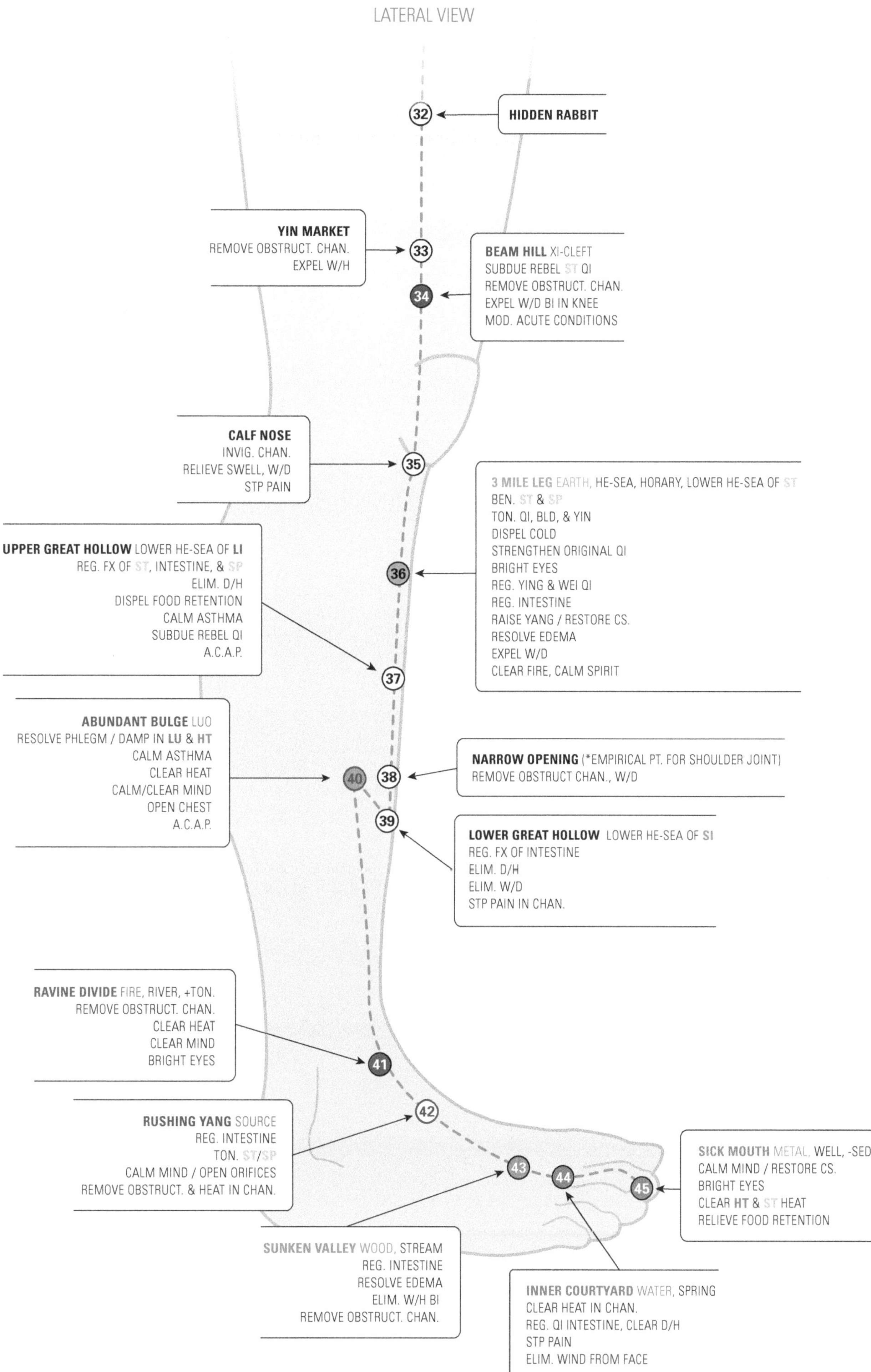
LATERAL VIEW
32
HIDDEN RABBIT
YIN MARKET
REMOVE OBSTRUCT. CHAN.
EXPEL W/H
33
BEAM HILL XI-CLEFT
SUBDUE REBEL ST QI
REMOVE OBSTRUCT. CHAN.
EXPEL W/D BI IN KNEE
MOD. ACUTE CONDITIONS
34
CALF NOSE
INVIG. CHAN.
RELIEVE SWELL, W/D
STP PAIN
35
3 MILE LEG EARTH, HE-SEA, HORARY, LOWER HE-SEA OF ST
BEN. ST & SP
TON. QI, BLD, & YIN
DISPEL COLD
STRENGTHEN ORIGINAL QI
BRIGHT EYES
REG. YING & WEI QI
REG. INTESTINE
RAISE YANG / RESTORE CS.
RESOLVE EDEMA
EXPEL W/D
CLEAR FIRE, CALM SPIRIT
36
UPPER GREAT HOLLOW LOWER HE-SEA OF LI
REG. FX OF ST, INTESTINE, & SP
ELIM. D/H
DISPEL FOOD RETENTION
CALM ASTHMA
SUBDUE REBEL QI
A.C.A.P.
37
ABUNDANT BULGE LUO
RESOLVE PHLEGM / DAMP IN LU & HT
CALM ASTHMA
CLEAR HEAT
CALM/CLEAR MIND
OPEN CHEST
A.C.A.P.
40
38
NARROW OPENING (*EMPIRICAL PT. FOR SHOULDER JOINT)
REMOVE OBSTRUCT CHAN., W/D
39
LOWER GREAT HOLLOW LOWER HE-SEA OF SI
REG. FX OF INTESTINE
ELIM. D/H
ELIM. W/D
STP PAIN IN CHAN.
RAVINE DIVIDE FIRE, RIVER, +TON.
REMOVE OBSTRUCT. CHAN.
CLEAR HEAT
CLEAR MIND
BRIGHT EYES
41
RUSHING YANG SOURCE
REG. INTESTINE
TON. ST/SP
CALM MIND / OPEN ORIFICES
REMOVE OBSTRUCT. & HEAT IN CHAN.
42
43
44
45
SICK MOUTH METAL, WELL, -SED.
CALM MIND / RESTORE CS.
BRIGHT EYES
CLEAR HT & ST HEAT
RELIEVE FOOD RETENTION
SUNKEN VALLEY WOOD, STREAM
REG. INTESTINE
RESOLVE EDEMA
ELIM. W/H BI
REMOVE OBSTRUCT. CHAN.
INNER COURTYARD WATER, SPRING
CLEAR HEAT IN CHAN.
REG. QI INTESTINE, CLEAR D/H
STP PAIN
ELIM. WIND FROM FACE

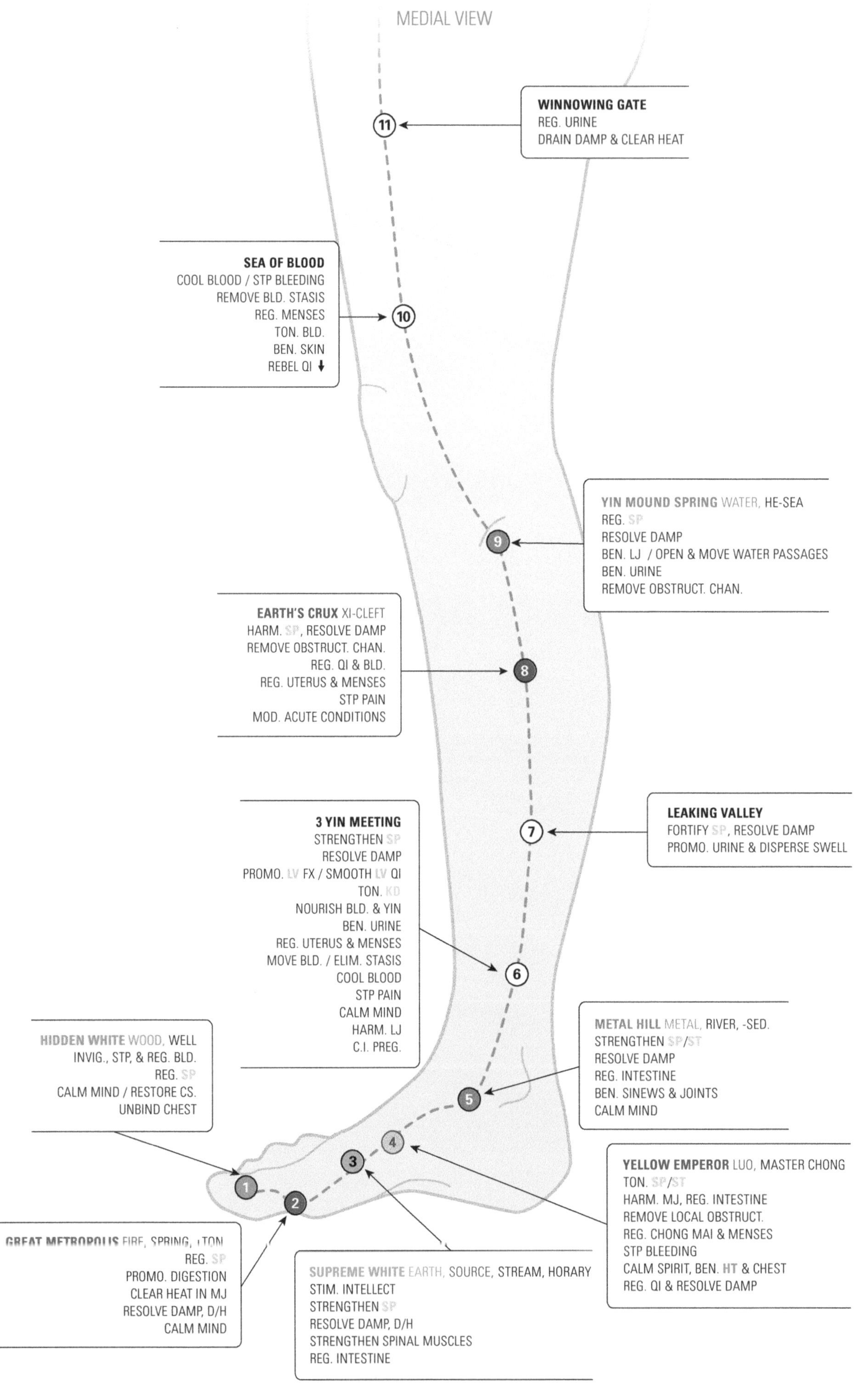
MEDIAL VIEW
WINNOWING GATE
REG. URINE
DRAIN DAMP & CLEAR HEAT
11
SEA OF BLOOD
COOL BLOOD / STP BLEEDING
REMOVE BLD. STASIS
REG. MENSES
TON. BLD.
BEN. SKIN
REBEL QI ↓
10
YIN MOUND SPRING WATER, HE-SEA
REG. SP
RESOLVE DAMP
BEN. LJ / OPEN & MOVE WATER PASSAGES
BEN. URINE
REMOVE OBSTRUCT. CHAN.
9
EARTH'S CRUX XI-CLEFT
HARM. SP, RESOLVE DAMP
REMOVE OBSTRUCT. CHAN.
REG. QI & BLD.
REG. UTERUS & MENSES
STP PAIN
MOD. ACUTE CONDITIONS
8
LEAKING VALLEY
FORTIFY SP, RESOLVE DAMP
PROMO. URINE & DISPERSE SWELL
7
3 YIN MEETING
STRENGTHEN SP
RESOLVE DAMP
PROMO. LV FX / SMOOTH LV QI
TON. KD
NOURISH BLD. & YIN
BEN. URINE
REG. UTERUS & MENSES
MOVE BLD. / ELIM. STASIS
COOL BLOOD
STP PAIN
CALM MIND
HARM. LJ
C.I. PREG.
6
METAL HILL METAL, RIVER, -SED.
STRENGTHEN SP/ST
RESOLVE DAMP
REG. INTESTINE
BEN. SINEWS & JOINTS
CALM MIND
5
HIDDEN WHITE WOOD, WELL
INVIG., STP, & REG. BLD.
REG. SP
CALM MIND / RESTORE CS.
UNBIND CHEST
4
3
1
2
YELLOW EMPEROR LUO, MASTER CHONG
TON. SP/ST
HARM. MJ, REG. INTESTINE
REMOVE LOCAL OBSTRUCT.
REG. CHONG MAI & MENSES
STP BLEEDING
CALM SPIRIT, BEN. HT & CHEST
REG. QI & RESOLVE DAMP
GREAT METROPOLIS FIRE, SPRING, ↑TON
REG. SP
PROMO. DIGESTION
CLEAR HEAT IN MJ
RESOLVE DAMP, D/H
CALM MIND
SUPREME WHITE EARTH, SOURCE, STREAM, HORARY
STIM. INTELLECT
STRENGTHEN SP
RESOLVE DAMP, D/H
STRENGTHEN SPINAL MUSCLES
REG. INTESTINE

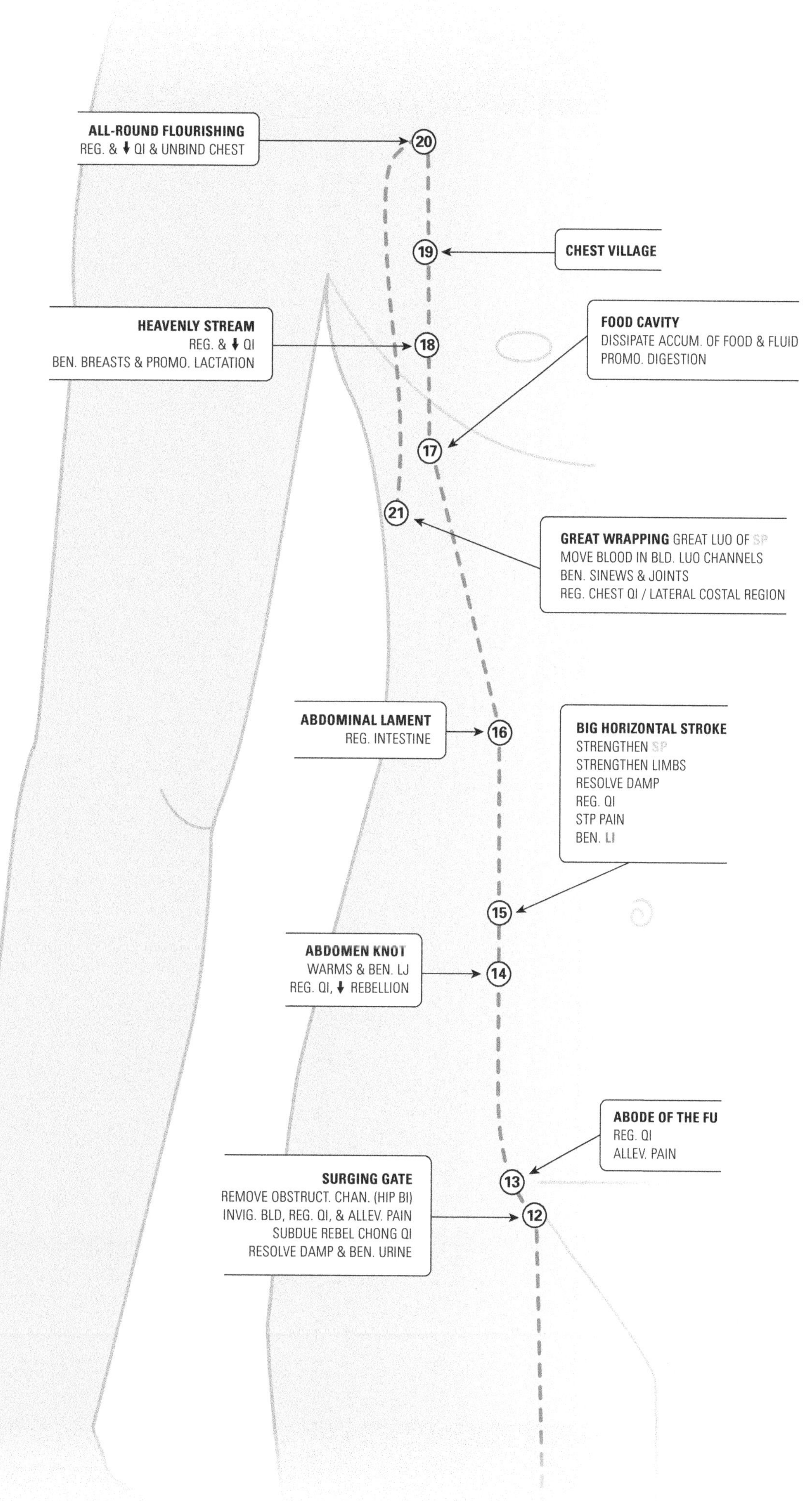
ALL-ROUND FLOURISHING
REG. & ↓ QI & UNBIND CHEST
20
CHEST VILLAGE
19
HEAVENLY STREAM
REG. & ↓ QI
BEN. BREASTS & PROMO. LACTATION
18
FOOD CAVITY
DISSIPATE ACCUM. OF FOOD & FLUID
PROMO. DIGESTION
17
21
GREAT WRAPPING GREAT LUO OF SP
MOVE BLOOD IN BLD. LUO CHANNELS
BEN. SINEWS & JOINTS
REG. CHEST QI / LATERAL COSTAL REGION
ABDOMINAL LAMENT
REG. INTESTINE
16
BIG HORIZONTAL STROKE
STRENGTHEN SP
STRENGTHEN LIMBS
RESOLVE DAMP
REG. QI
STP PAIN
BEN. LI
15
ABDOMEN KNOT
WARMS & BEN. LJ
REG. QI, ↓ REBELLION
14
ABODE OF THE FU
REG. QI
ALLEV. PAIN
13
SURGING GATE
REMOVE OBSTRUCT. CHAN. (HIP BI)
INVIG. BLD, REG. QI, & ALLEV. PAIN
SUBDUE REBEL CHONG QI
RESOLVE DAMP & BEN. URINE
12

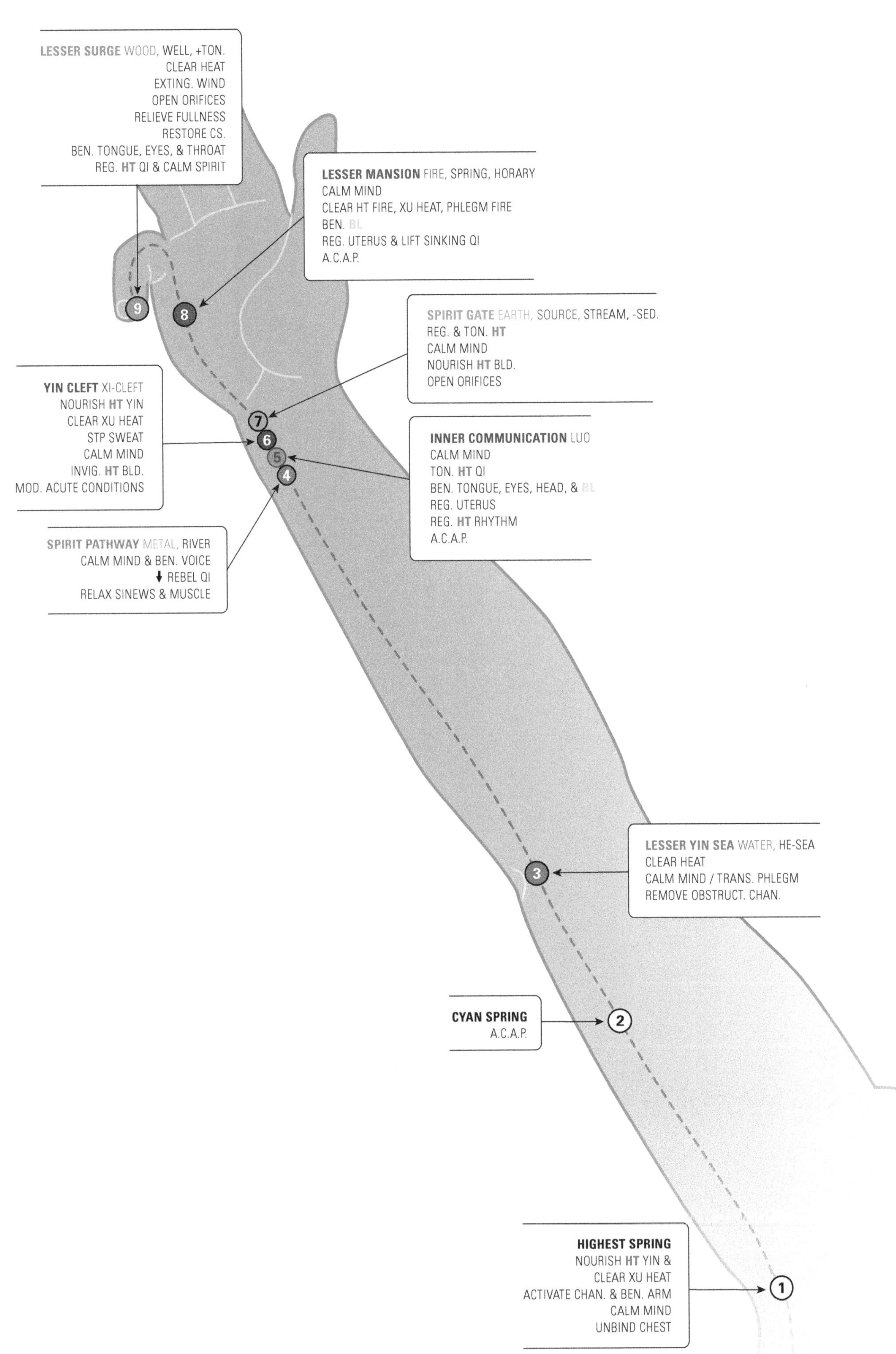
LESSER SURGE WOOD, WELL, +TON.
CLEAR HEAT
EXTING. WIND
OPEN ORIFICES
RELIEVE FULLNESS
RESTORE CS.
BEN. TONGUE, EYES, & THROAT
REG. HT QI & CALM SPIRIT
LESSER MANSION FIRE, SPRING, HORARY
CALM MIND
CLEAR HT FIRE, XU HEAT, PHLEGM FIRE
BEN. BL
REG. UTERUS & LIFT SINKING QI
A.C.A.P.
9
8
SPIRIT GATE EARTH, SOURCE, STREAM, -SED.
REG. & TON. HT
CALM MIND
NOURISH HT BLD.
OPEN ORIFICES
YIN CLEFT XI-CLEFT
NOURISH HT YIN
CLEAR XU HEAT
STP SWEAT
CALM MIND
INVIG. HT BLD.
MOD. ACUTE CONDITIONS
7
6
5
4
INNER COMMUNICATION LUO
CALM MIND
TON. HT QI
BEN. TONGUE, EYES, HEAD, & BL
REG. UTERUS
REG. HT RHYTHM
A.C.A.P.
SPIRIT PATHWAY METAL, RIVER
CALM MIND & BEN. VOICE
⬇ REBEL QI
RELAX SINEWS & MUSCLE
3
LESSER YIN SEA WATER, HE-SEA
CLEAR HEAT
CALM MIND / TRANS. PHLEGM
REMOVE OBSTRUCT. CHAN.
CYAN SPRING
A.C.A.P.
2
HIGHEST SPRING
NOURISH HT YIN &
CLEAR XU HEAT
ACTIVATE CHAN. & BEN. ARM
CALM MIND
UNBIND CHEST
1

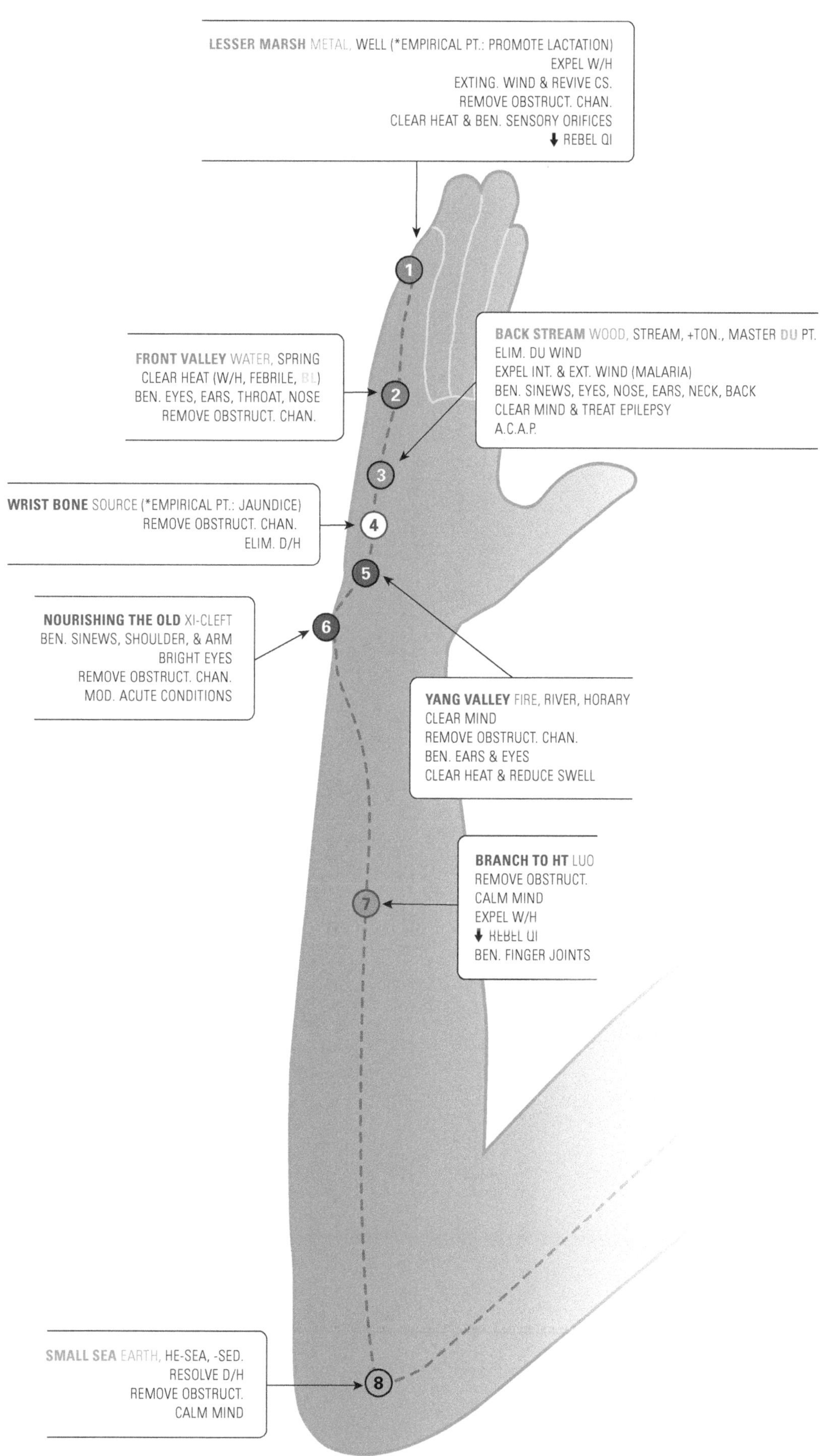
LESSER MARSH METAL, WELL (*EMPIRICAL PT.: PROMOTE LACTATION)
EXPEL W/H
EXTING. WIND & REVIVE CS.
REMOVE OBSTRUCT. CHAN.
CLEAR HEAT & BEN. SENSORY ORIFICES
⬇ REBEL QI
1
FRONT VALLEY WATER, SPRING
CLEAR HEAT (W/H, FEBRILE, BL)
BEN. EYES, EARS, THROAT, NOSE
REMOVE OBSTRUCT. CHAN.
2
BACK STREAM WOOD, STREAM, +TON., MASTER DU PT.
ELIM. DU WIND
EXPEL INT. & EXT. WIND (MALARIA)
BEN. SINEWS, EYES, NOSE, EARS, NECK, BACK
CLEAR MIND & TREAT EPILEPSY
A.C.A.P.
3
WRIST BONE SOURCE (*EMPIRICAL PT.: JAUNDICE)
REMOVE OBSTRUCT. CHAN.
ELIM. D/H
4
5
NOURISHING THE OLD XI-CLEFT
BEN. SINEWS, SHOULDER, & ARM
BRIGHT EYES
REMOVE OBSTRUCT. CHAN.
MOD. ACUTE CONDITIONS
6
YANG VALLEY FIRE, RIVER, HORARY
CLEAR MIND
REMOVE OBSTRUCT. CHAN.
BEN. EARS & EYES
CLEAR HEAT & REDUCE SWELL
BRANCH TO HT LUO
REMOVE OBSTRUCT.
CALM MIND
EXPEL W/H
⬇ REBEL QI
BEN. FINGER JOINTS
7
SMALL SEA EARTH, HE-SEA, -SED.
RESOLVE D/H
REMOVE OBSTRUCT.
CALM MIND
8

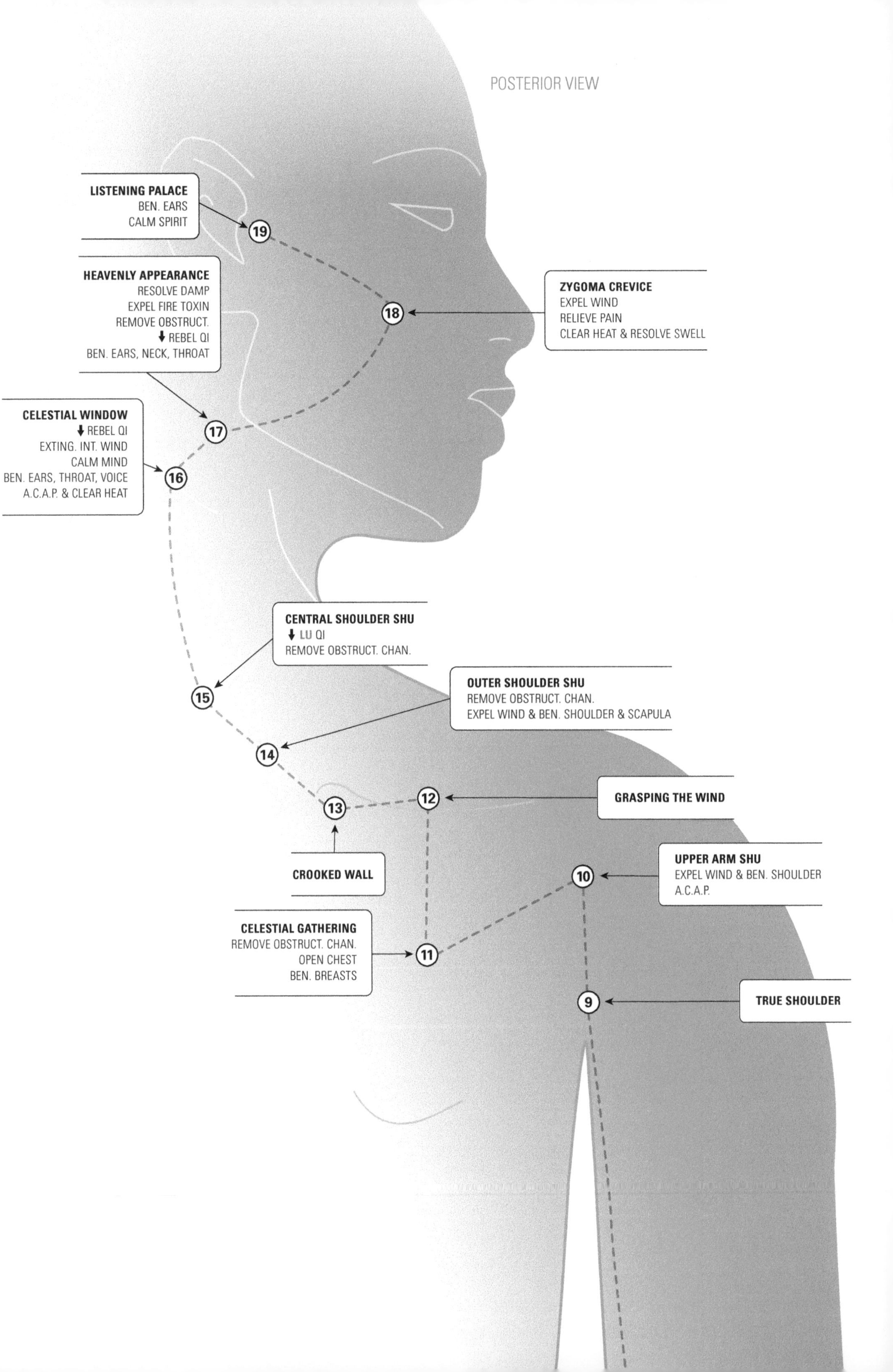

POSTERIOR VIEW

LISTENING PALACE
BEN. EARS
CALM SPIRIT
19

HEAVENLY APPEARANCE
RESOLVE DAMP
EXPEL FIRE TOXIN
REMOVE OBSTRUCT.
↓ REBEL QI
BEN. EARS, NECK, THROAT
17

ZYGOMA CREVICE
EXPEL WIND
RELIEVE PAIN
CLEAR HEAT & RESOLVE SWELL
18

CELESTIAL WINDOW
↓ REBEL QI
EXTING. INT. WIND
CALM MIND
BEN. EARS, THROAT, VOICE
A.C.A.P. & CLEAR HEAT
16

CENTRAL SHOULDER SHU
↓ LU QI
REMOVE OBSTRUCT. CHAN.
15

OUTER SHOULDER SHU
REMOVE OBSTRUCT. CHAN.
EXPEL WIND & BEN. SHOULDER & SCAPULA
14

GRASPING THE WIND
12

CROOKED WALL
13

UPPER ARM SHU
EXPEL WIND & BEN. SHOULDER
A.C.A.P.
10

CELESTIAL GATHERING
REMOVE OBSTRUCT. CHAN.
OPEN CHEST
BEN. BREASTS
11

TRUE SHOULDER
9

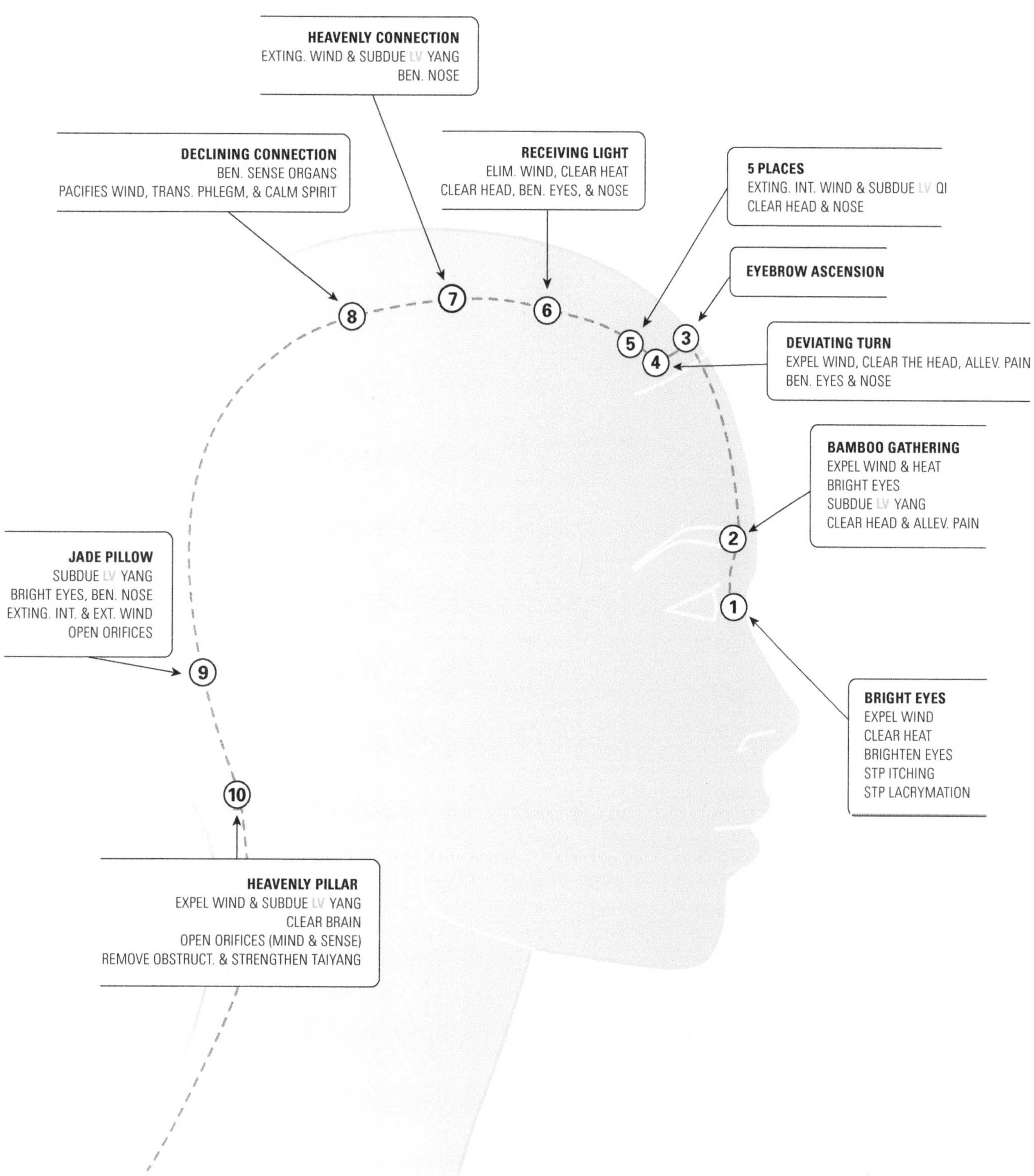
HEAVENLY CONNECTION
EXTING. WIND & SUBDUE LV YANG
BEN. NOSE
DECLINING CONNECTION
BEN. SENSE ORGANS
PACIFIES WIND, TRANS. PHLEGM, & CALM SPIRIT
RECEIVING LIGHT
ELIM. WIND, CLEAR HEAT
CLEAR HEAD, BEN. EYES, & NOSE
5 PLACES
EXTING. INT. WIND & SUBDUE LV QI
CLEAR HEAD & NOSE
EYEBROW ASCENSION
DEVIATING TURN
EXPEL WIND, CLEAR THE HEAD, ALLEV. PAIN
BEN. EYES & NOSE
BAMBOO GATHERING
EXPEL WIND & HEAT
BRIGHT EYES
SUBDUE LV YANG
CLEAR HEAD & ALLEV. PAIN
JADE PILLOW
SUBDUE LV YANG
BRIGHT EYES, BEN. NOSE
EXTING. INT. & EXT. WIND
OPEN ORIFICES
BRIGHT EYES
EXPEL WIND
CLEAR HEAT
BRIGHTEN EYES
STP ITCHING
STP LACRYMATION
HEAVENLY PILLAR
EXPEL WIND & SUBDUE LV YANG
CLEAR BRAIN
OPEN ORIFICES (MIND & SENSE)
REMOVE OBSTRUCT. & STRENGTHEN TAIYANG
1
2
3
4
5
6
7
8
9
10

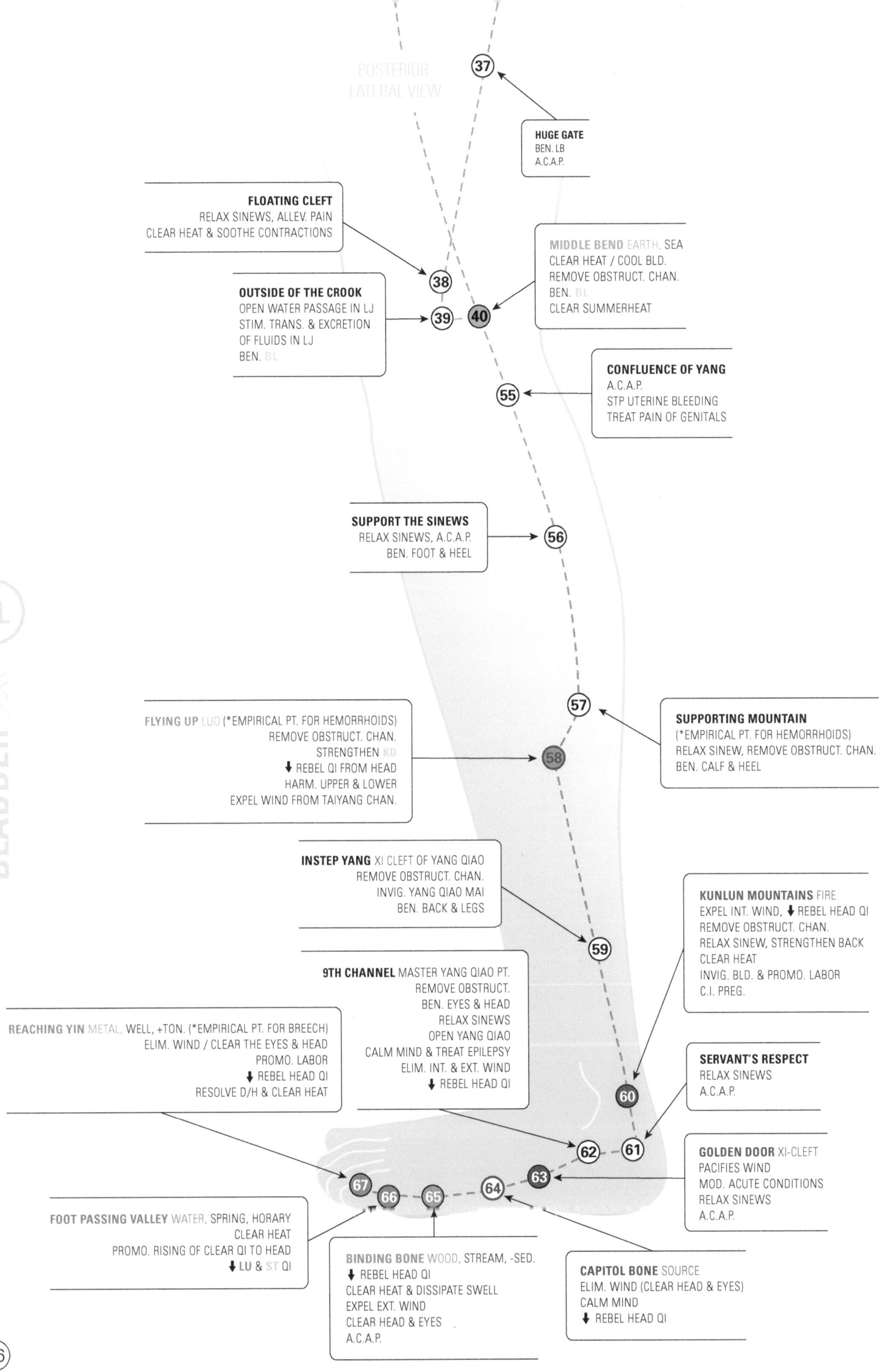

POSTERIOR
LATERAL VIEW

HUGE GATE
BEN. LB
A.C.A.P.

37

FLOATING CLEFT
RELAX SINEWS, ALLEV. PAIN
CLEAR HEAT & SOOTHE CONTRACTIONS

38

MIDDLE BEND EARTH, SEA
CLEAR HEAT / COOL BLD.
REMOVE OBSTRUCT. CHAN.
BEN. BL
CLEAR SUMMERHEAT

40

OUTSIDE OF THE CROOK
OPEN WATER PASSAGE IN LJ
STIM. TRANS. & EXCRETION
OF FLUIDS IN LJ
BEN. BL

39

CONFLUENCE OF YANG
A.C.A.P.
STP UTERINE BLEEDING
TREAT PAIN OF GENITALS

55

SUPPORT THE SINEWS
RELAX SINEWS, A.C.A.P.
BEN. FOOT & HEEL

56

SUPPORTING MOUNTAIN
(*EMPIRICAL PT. FOR HEMORRHOIDS)
RELAX SINEW, REMOVE OBSTRUCT. CHAN.
BEN. CALF & HEEL

57

FLYING UP LUO (*EMPIRICAL PT. FOR HEMORRHOIDS)
REMOVE OBSTRUCT. CHAN.
STRENGTHEN KD
⬇ REBEL QI FROM HEAD
HARM. UPPER & LOWER
EXPEL WIND FROM TAIYANG CHAN.

58

INSTEP YANG XI CLEFT OF YANG QIAO
REMOVE OBSTRUCT. CHAN.
INVIG. YANG QIAO MAI
BEN. BACK & LEGS

59

KUNLUN MOUNTAINS FIRE
EXPEL INT. WIND, ⬇ REBEL HEAD QI
REMOVE OBSTRUCT. CHAN.
RELAX SINEW, STRENGTHEN BACK
CLEAR HEAT
INVIG. BLD. & PROMO. LABOR
C.I. PREG.

60

SERVANT'S RESPECT
RELAX SINEWS
A.C.A.P.

61

9TH CHANNEL MASTER YANG QIAO PT.
REMOVE OBSTRUCT.
BEN. EYES & HEAD
RELAX SINEWS
OPEN YANG QIAO
CALM MIND & TREAT EPILEPSY
ELIM. INT. & EXT. WIND
⬇ REBEL HEAD QI

62

GOLDEN DOOR XI-CLEFT
PACIFIES WIND
MOD. ACUTE CONDITIONS
RELAX SINEWS
A.C.A.P.

63

CAPITOL BONE SOURCE
ELIM. WIND (CLEAR HEAD & EYES)
CALM MIND
⬇ REBEL HEAD QI

64

BINDING BONE WOOD, STREAM, -SED.
⬇ REBEL HEAD QI
CLEAR HEAT & DISSIPATE SWELL
EXPEL EXT. WIND
CLEAR HEAD & EYES
A.C.A.P.

65

FOOT PASSING VALLEY WATER, SPRING, HORARY
CLEAR HEAT
PROMO. RISING OF CLEAR QI TO HEAD
⬇ **LU** & **ST** QI

66

REACHING YIN METAL, WELL, +TON. (*EMPIRICAL PT. FOR BREECH)
ELIM. WIND / CLEAR THE EYES & HEAD
PROMO. LABOR
⬇ REBEL HEAD QI
RESOLVE D/H & CLEAR HEAT

67

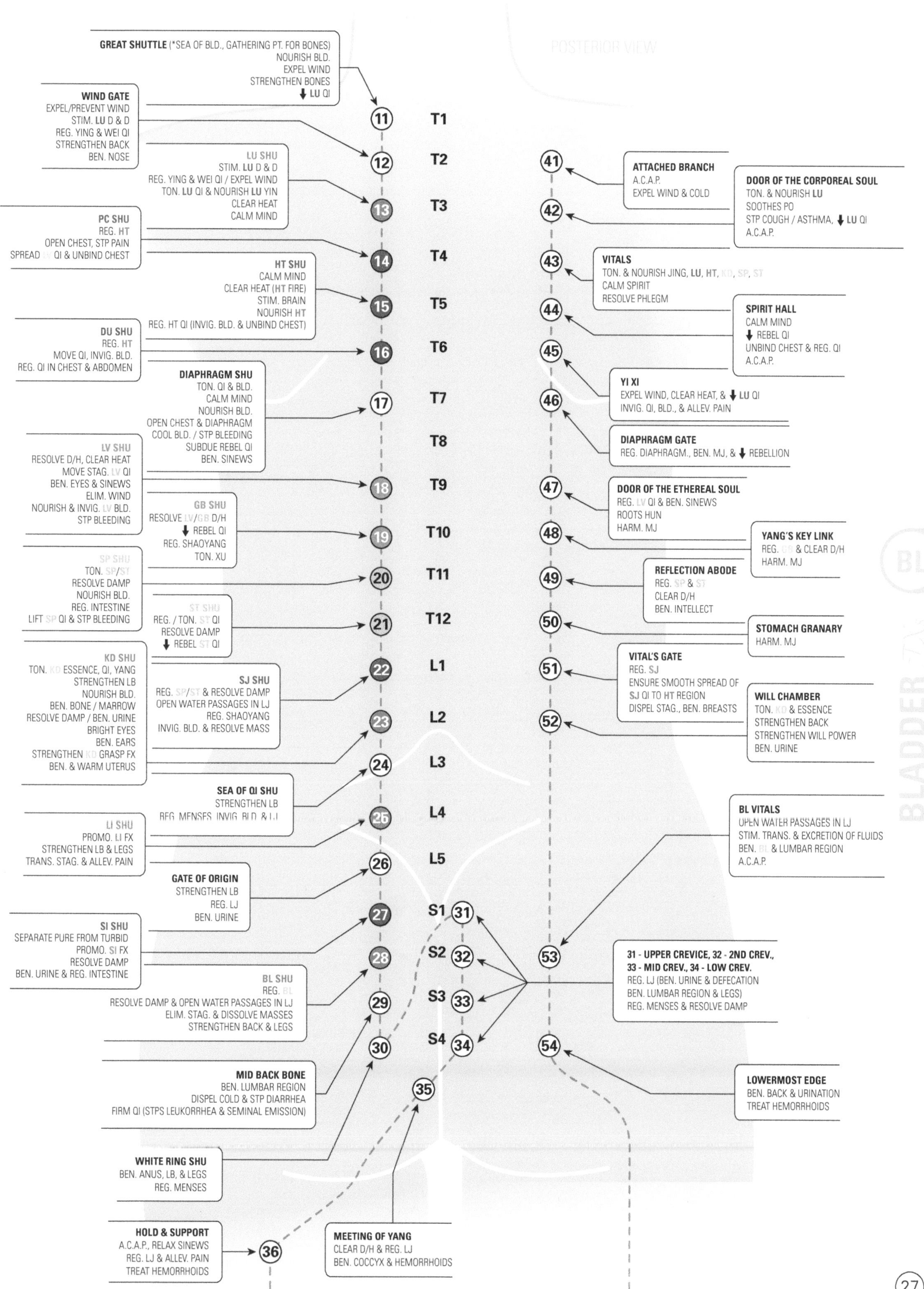

POSTERIOR VIEW
GREAT SHUTTLE (*SEA OF BLD., GATHERING PT. FOR BONES)
NOURISH BLD.
EXPEL WIND
STRENGTHEN BONES
↓ LU QI
WIND GATE
EXPEL/PREVENT WIND
STIM. LU D & D
REG. YING & WEI QI
STRENGTHEN BACK
BEN. NOSE
LU SHU
STIM. LU D & D
REG. YING & WEI QI / EXPEL WIND
TON. LU QI & NOURISH LU YIN
CLEAR HEAT
CALM MIND
PC SHU
REG. HT
OPEN CHEST, STP PAIN
SPREAD LV QI & UNBIND CHEST
HT SHU
CALM MIND
CLEAR HEAT (HT FIRE)
STIM. BRAIN
NOURISH HT
REG. HT QI (INVIG. BLD. & UNBIND CHEST)
DU SHU
REG. HT
MOVE QI, INVIG. BLD.
REG. QI IN CHEST & ABDOMEN
DIAPHRAGM SHU
TON. QI & BLD.
CALM MIND
NOURISH BLD.
OPEN CHEST & DIAPHRAGM
COOL BLD. / STP BLEEDING
SUBDUE REBEL QI
BEN. SINEWS
LV SHU
RESOLVE D/H, CLEAR HEAT
MOVE STAG. LV QI
BEN. EYES & SINEWS
ELIM. WIND
NOURISH & INVIG. LV BLD.
STP BLEEDING
GB SHU
RESOLVE LV/GB D/H
↓ REBEL QI
REG. SHAOYANG
TON. XU
SP SHU
TON. SP/ST
RESOLVE DAMP
NOURISH BLD.
REG. INTESTINE
LIFT SP QI & STP BLEEDING
ST SHU
REG. / TON. ST QI
RESOLVE DAMP
↓ REBEL ST QI
KD SHU
TON. KD ESSENCE, QI, YANG
STRENGTHEN LB
NOURISH BLD.
BEN. BONE / MARROW
RESOLVE DAMP / BEN. URINE
BRIGHT EYES
BEN. EARS
STRENGTHEN KD GRASP FX
BEN. & WARM UTERUS
SJ SHU
REG. SP/ST & RESOLVE DAMP
OPEN WATER PASSAGES IN LJ
REG. SHAOYANG
INVIG. BLD. & RESOLVE MASS
SEA OF QI SHU
STRENGTHEN LB
REG. MENSES, INVIG. BLD. & LJ
LI SHU
PROMO. LI FX
STRENGTHEN LB & LEGS
TRANS. STAG. & ALLEV. PAIN
GATE OF ORIGIN
STRENGTHEN LB
REG. LJ
BEN. URINE
SI SHU
SEPARATE PURE FROM TURBID
PROMO. SI FX
RESOLVE DAMP
BEN. URINE & REG. INTESTINE
BL SHU
REG. BL
RESOLVE DAMP & OPEN WATER PASSAGES IN LJ
ELIM. STAG. & DISSOLVE MASSES
STRENGTHEN BACK & LEGS
MID BACK BONE
BEN. LUMBAR REGION
DISPEL COLD & STP DIARRHEA
FIRM QI (STPS LEUKORRHEA & SEMINAL EMISSION)
WHITE RING SHU
BEN. ANUS, LB, & LEGS
REG. MENSES
HOLD & SUPPORT
A.C.A.P., RELAX SINEWS
REG. LJ & ALLEV. PAIN
TREAT HEMORRHOIDS
MEETING OF YANG
CLEAR D/H & REG. LJ
BEN. COCCYX & HEMORRHOIDS
11
12
13
14
15
16
17
18
19
20
21
22
23
24
25
26
27
28
29
30
31
32
33
34
35
36
T1
T2
T3
T4
T5
T6
T7
T8
T9
T10
T11
T12
L1
L2
L3
L4
L5
S1
S2
S3
S4
41
42
43
44
45
46
47
48
49
50
51
52
53
54
ATTACHED BRANCH
A.C.A.P.
EXPEL WIND & COLD
DOOR OF THE CORPOREAL SOUL
TON. & NOURISH LU
SOOTHES PO
STP COUGH / ASTHMA, ↓ LU QI
A.C.A.P.
VITALS
TON. & NOURISH JING, LU, HT, KD, SP, ST
CALM SPIRIT
RESOLVE PHLEGM
SPIRIT HALL
CALM MIND
↓ REBEL QI
UNBIND CHEST & REG. QI
A.C.A.P.
YI XI
EXPEL WIND, CLEAR HEAT, & ↓ LU QI
INVIG. QI, BLD., & ALLEV. PAIN
DIAPHRAGM GATE
REG. DIAPHRAGM., BEN. MJ, & ↓ REBELLION
DOOR OF THE ETHEREAL SOUL
REG. LV QI & BEN. SINEWS
ROOTS HUN
HARM. MJ
YANG'S KEY LINK
REG. GB & CLEAR D/H
HARM. MJ
REFLECTION ABODE
REG. SP & ST
CLEAR D/H
BEN. INTELLECT
STOMACH GRANARY
HARM. MJ
VITAL'S GATE
REG. SJ
ENSURE SMOOTH SPREAD OF
SJ QI TO HT REGION
DISPEL STAG., BEN. BREASTS
WILL CHAMBER
TON. KD & ESSENCE
STRENGTHEN BACK
STRENGTHEN WILL POWER
BEN. URINE
BL VITALS
OPEN WATER PASSAGES IN LJ
STIM. TRANS. & EXCRETION OF FLUIDS
BEN. BL & LUMBAR REGION
A.C.A.P.
31 - UPPER CREVICE, 32 - 2ND CREV.,
33 - MID CREV., 34 - LOW CREV.
REG. LJ (BEN. URINE & DEFECATION
BEN. LUMBAR REGION & LEGS)
REG. MENSES & RESOLVE DAMP
LOWERMOST EDGE
BEN. BACK & URINATION
TREAT HEMORRHOIDS
BL
BLADDER

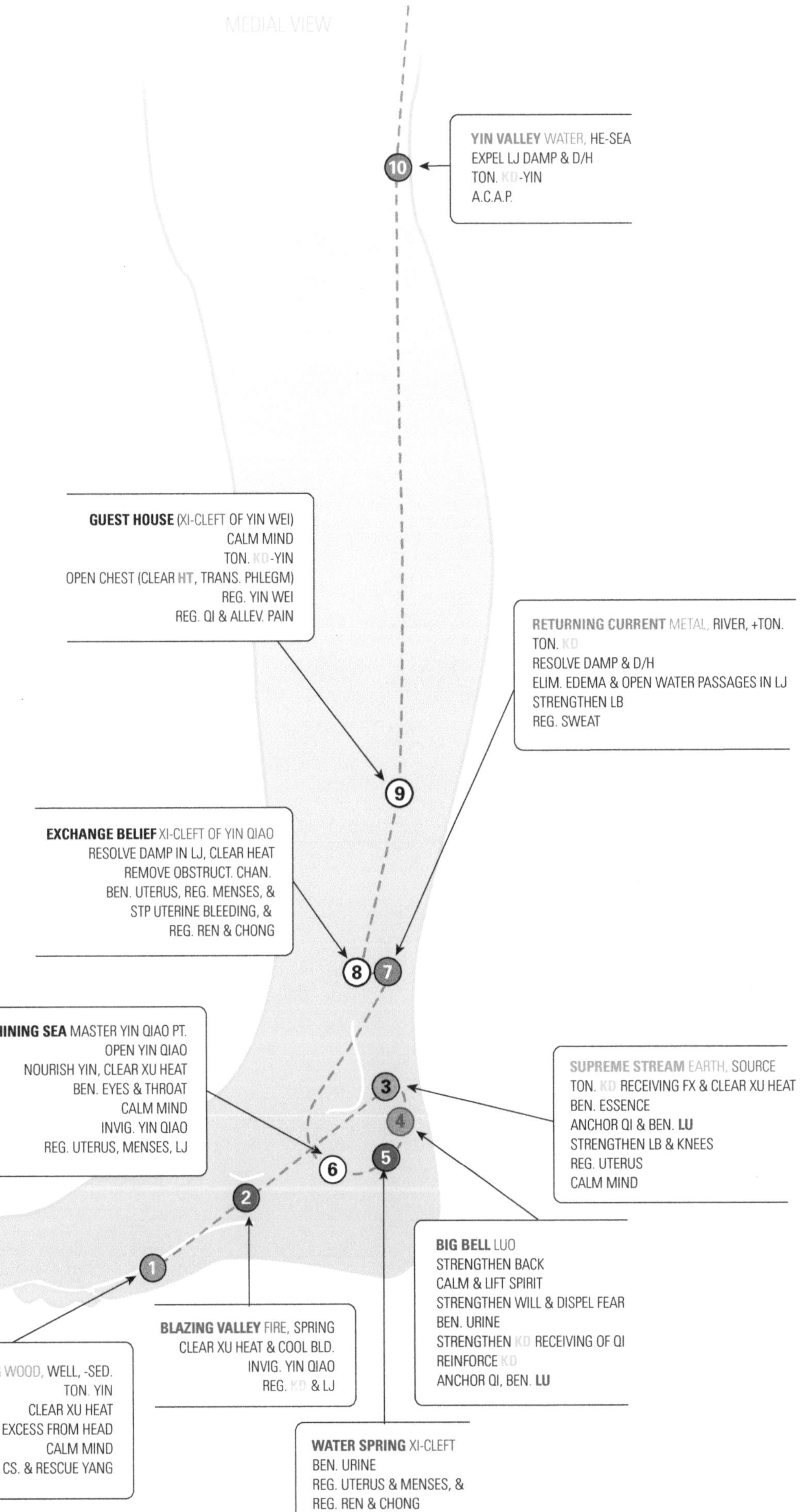

MEDIAL VIEW
YIN VALLEY WATER, HE-SEA
EXPEL LJ DAMP & D/H
TON. KD-YIN
A.C.A.P.
10
GUEST HOUSE (XI-CLEFT OF YIN WEI)
CALM MIND
TON. KD-YIN
OPEN CHEST (CLEAR HT, TRANS. PHLEGM)
REG. YIN WEI
REG. QI & ALLEV. PAIN
RETURNING CURRENT METAL, RIVER, +TON.
TON. KD
RESOLVE DAMP & D/H
ELIM. EDEMA & OPEN WATER PASSAGES IN LJ
STRENGTHEN LB
REG. SWEAT
9
EXCHANGE BELIEF XI-CLEFT OF YIN QIAO
RESOLVE DAMP IN LJ, CLEAR HEAT
REMOVE OBSTRUCT. CHAN.
BEN. UTERUS, REG. MENSES, &
STP UTERINE BLEEDING, &
REG. REN & CHONG
8
7
SHINING SEA MASTER YIN QIAO PT.
OPEN YIN QIAO
NOURISH YIN, CLEAR XU HEAT
BEN. EYES & THROAT
CALM MIND
INVIG. YIN QIAO
REG. UTERUS, MENSES, LJ
3
4
5
6
2
1
SUPREME STREAM EARTH, SOURCE
TON. KD RECEIVING FX & CLEAR XU HEAT
BEN. ESSENCE
ANCHOR QI & BEN. LU
STRENGTHEN LB & KNEES
REG. UTERUS
CALM MIND
BIG BELL LUO
STRENGTHEN BACK
CALM & LIFT SPIRIT
STRENGTHEN WILL & DISPEL FEAR
BEN. URINE
STRENGTHEN KD RECEIVING OF QI
REINFORCE KD
ANCHOR QI, BEN. LU
BLAZING VALLEY FIRE, SPRING
CLEAR XU HEAT & COOL BLD.
INVIG. YIN QIAO
REG. KD & LJ
GUSHING SPRING WOOD, WELL, -SED.
TON. YIN
CLEAR XU HEAT
SUBDUE INT. WIND ⬇ EXCESS FROM HEAD
CALM MIND
RESTORE CS. & RESCUE YANG
WATER SPRING XI-CLEFT
BEN. URINE
REG. UTERUS & MENSES, &
REG. REN & CHONG

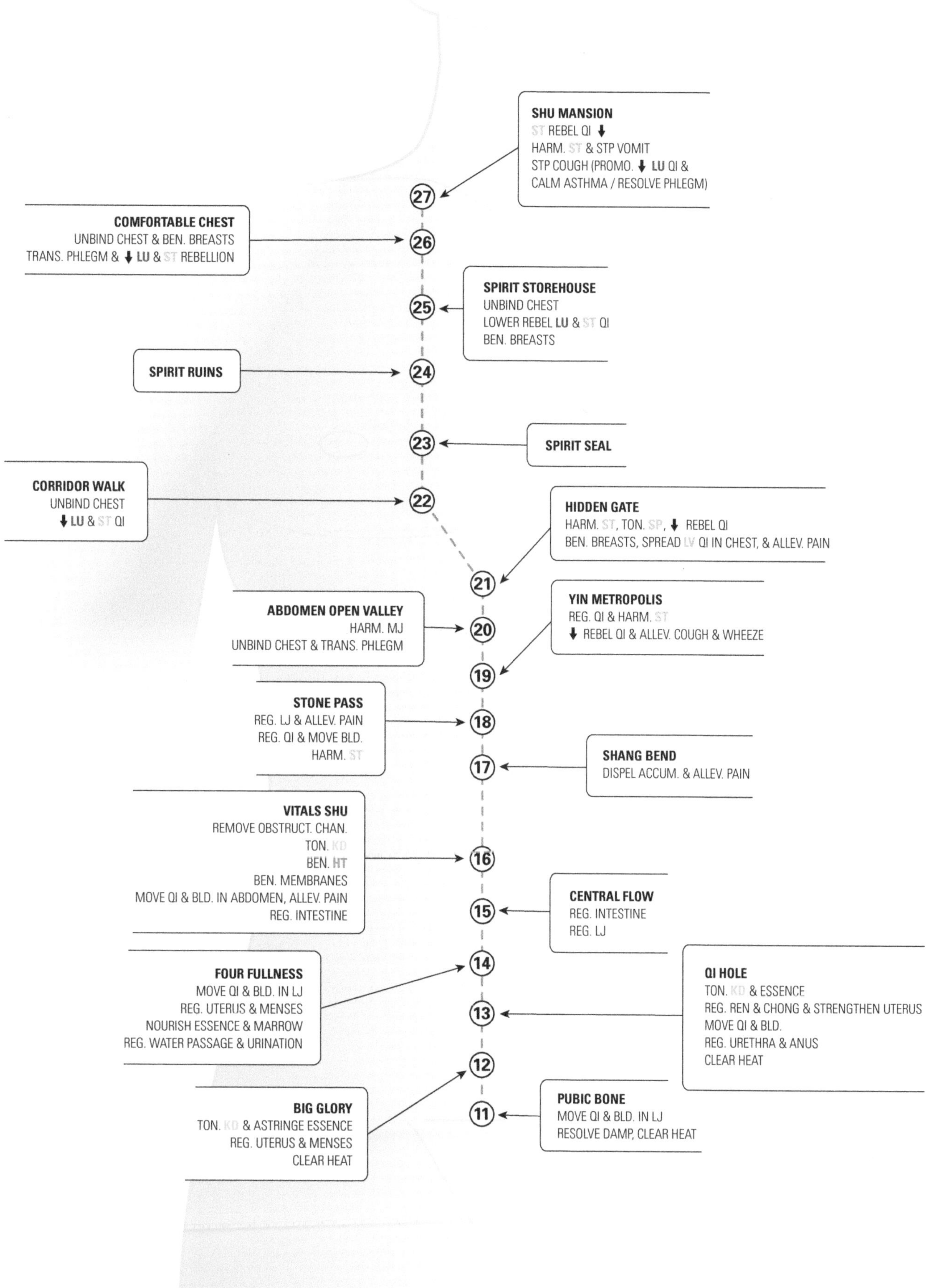

SHU MANSION
ST REBEL QI ↓
HARM. ST & STP VOMIT
STP COUGH (PROMO. ↓ LU QI &
CALM ASTHMA / RESOLVE PHLEGM)
27
COMFORTABLE CHEST
UNBIND CHEST & BEN. BREASTS
TRANS. PHLEGM & ↓ LU & ST REBELLION
26
SPIRIT STOREHOUSE
UNBIND CHEST
LOWER REBEL LU & ST QI
BEN. BREASTS
25
SPIRIT RUINS
24
SPIRIT SEAL
23
CORRIDOR WALK
UNBIND CHEST
↓ LU & ST QI
22
HIDDEN GATE
HARM. ST, TON. SP, ↓ REBEL QI
BEN. BREASTS, SPREAD LV QI IN CHEST, & ALLEV. PAIN
21
ABDOMEN OPEN VALLEY
HARM. MJ
UNBIND CHEST & TRANS. PHLEGM
20
YIN METROPOLIS
REG. QI & HARM. ST
↓ REBEL QI & ALLEV. COUGH & WHEEZE
19
STONE PASS
REG. LJ & ALLEV. PAIN
REG. QI & MOVE BLD.
HARM. ST
18
SHANG BEND
DISPEL ACCUM. & ALLEV. PAIN
17
VITALS SHU
REMOVE OBSTRUCT. CHAN.
TON. KD
BEN. HT
BEN. MEMBRANES
MOVE QI & BLD. IN ABDOMEN, ALLEV. PAIN
REG. INTESTINE
16
CENTRAL FLOW
REG. INTESTINE
REG. LJ
15
FOUR FULLNESS
MOVE QI & BLD. IN LJ
REG. UTERUS & MENSES
NOURISH ESSENCE & MARROW
REG. WATER PASSAGE & URINATION
14
QI HOLE
TON. KD & ESSENCE
REG. REN & CHONG & STRENGTHEN UTERUS
MOVE QI & BLD.
REG. URETHRA & ANUS
CLEAR HEAT
13
12
BIG GLORY
TON. KD & ASTRINGE ESSENCE
REG. UTERUS & MENSES
CLEAR HEAT
PUBIC BONE
MOVE QI & BLD. IN LJ
RESOLVE DAMP, CLEAR HEAT
11

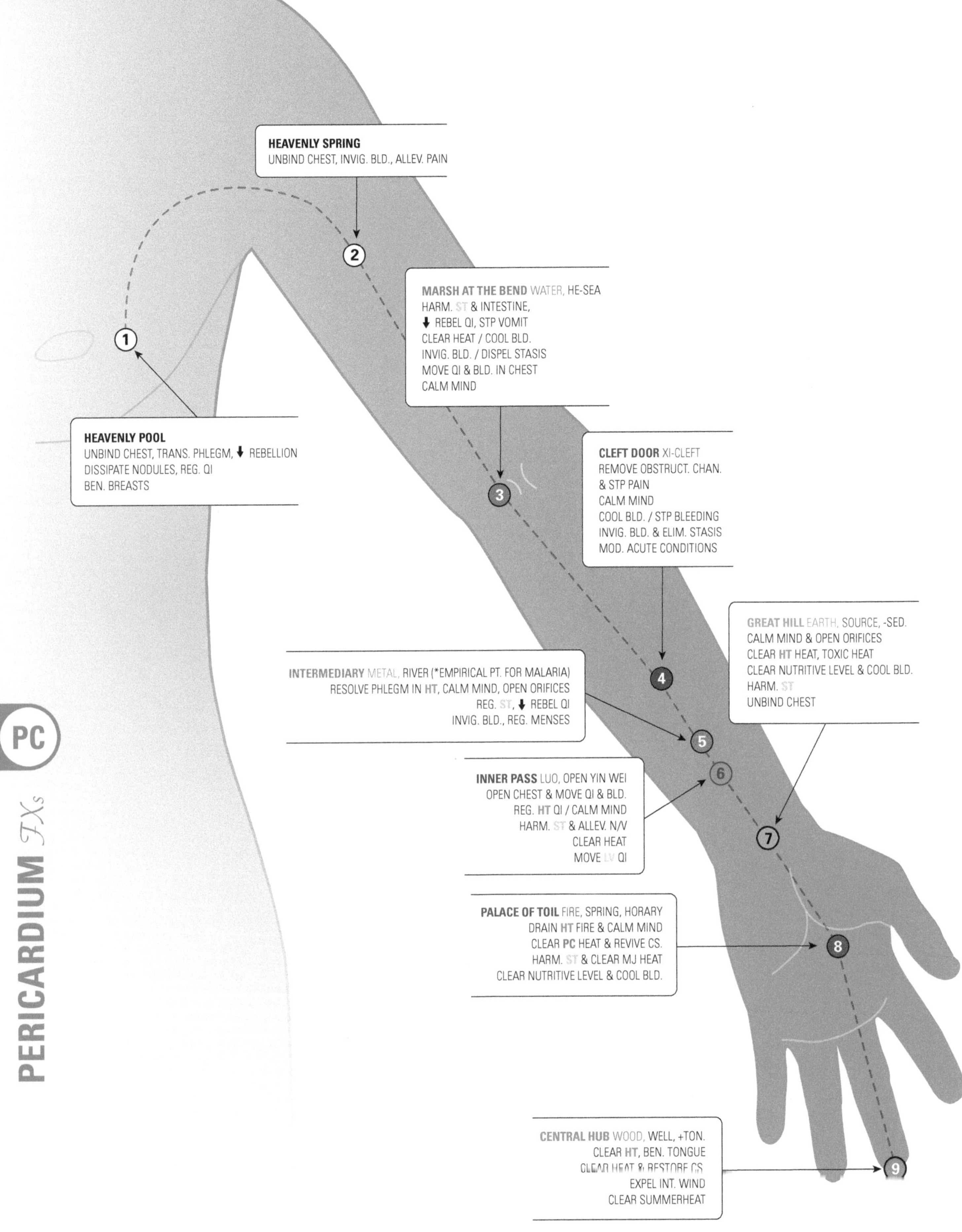
HEAVENLY SPRING
UNBIND CHEST, INVIG. BLD., ALLEV. PAIN
2
MARSH AT THE BEND WATER, HE-SEA
HARM. ST & INTESTINE,
⬇ REBEL QI, STP VOMIT
CLEAR HEAT / COOL BLD.
INVIG. BLD. / DISPEL STASIS
MOVE QI & BLD. IN CHEST
CALM MIND
1
HEAVENLY POOL
UNBIND CHEST, TRANS. PHLEGM, ⬇ REBELLION
DISSIPATE NODULES, REG. QI
BEN. BREASTS
CLEFT DOOR XI-CLEFT
REMOVE OBSTRUCT. CHAN.
& STP PAIN
CALM MIND
COOL BLD. / STP BLEEDING
INVIG. BLD. & ELIM. STASIS
MOD. ACUTE CONDITIONS
3
GREAT HILL EARTH, SOURCE, -SED.
CALM MIND & OPEN ORIFICES
CLEAR HT HEAT, TOXIC HEAT
CLEAR NUTRITIVE LEVEL & COOL BLD.
HARM. ST
UNBIND CHEST
INTERMEDIARY METAL, RIVER (*EMPIRICAL PT. FOR MALARIA)
RESOLVE PHLEGM IN HT, CALM MIND, OPEN ORIFICES
REG. ST, ⬇ REBEL QI
INVIG. BLD., REG. MENSES
4
5
6
INNER PASS LUO, OPEN YIN WEI
OPEN CHEST & MOVE QI & BLD.
REG. HT QI / CALM MIND
HARM. ST & ALLEV. N/V
CLEAR HEAT
MOVE LV QI
7
PALACE OF TOIL FIRE, SPRING, HORARY
DRAIN HT FIRE & CALM MIND
CLEAR PC HEAT & REVIVE CS.
HARM. ST & CLEAR MJ HEAT
CLEAR NUTRITIVE LEVEL & COOL BLD.
8
CENTRAL HUB WOOD, WELL, +TON.
CLEAR HT, BEN. TONGUE
CLEAR HEAT & RESTORE CS.
EXPEL INT. WIND
CLEAR SUMMERHEAT
9

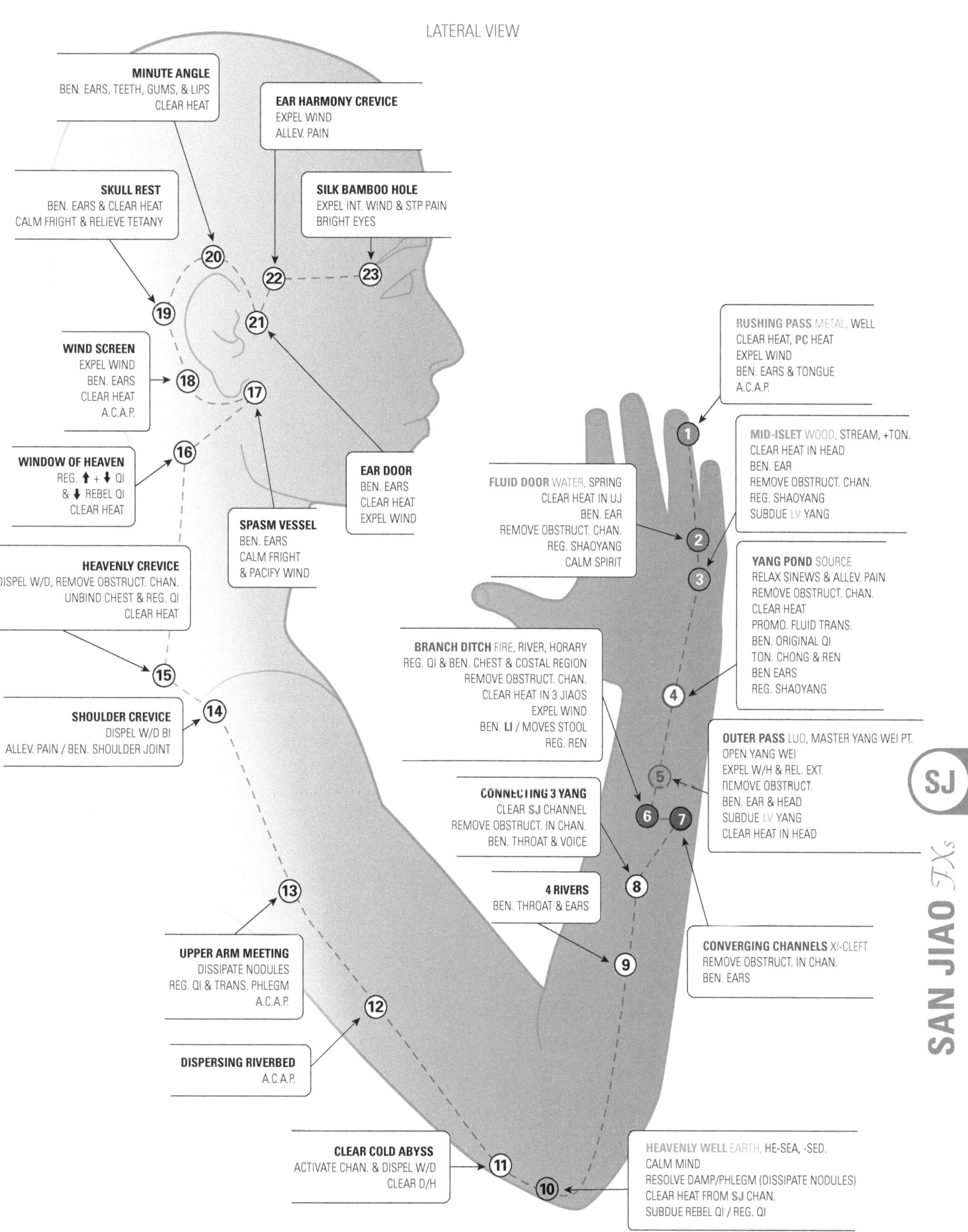
LATERAL VIEW
MINUTE ANGLE
BEN. EARS, TEETH, GUMS, & LIPS
CLEAR HEAT
EAR HARMONY CREVICE
EXPEL WIND
ALLEV. PAIN
SKULL REST
BEN. EARS & CLEAR HEAT
CALM FRIGHT & RELIEVE TETANY
SILK BAMBOO HOLE
EXPEL INT. WIND & STP PAIN
BRIGHT EYES
RUSHING PASS METAL, WELL
CLEAR HEAT, PC HEAT
EXPEL WIND
BEN. EARS & TONGUE
A.C.A.P.
WIND SCREEN
EXPEL WIND
BEN. EARS
CLEAR HEAT
A.C.A.P.
MID-ISLET WOOD, STREAM, +TON.
CLEAR HEAT IN HEAD
BEN. EAR
REMOVE OBSTRUCT. CHAN.
REG. SHAOYANG
SUBDUE LV YANG
WINDOW OF HEAVEN
REG. ⬆ + ⬇ QI
& ⬇ REBEL QI
CLEAR HEAT
EAR DOOR
BEN. EARS
CLEAR HEAT
EXPEL WIND
FLUID DOOR WATER, SPRING
CLEAR HEAT IN UJ
BEN. EAR
REMOVE OBSTRUCT. CHAN.
REG. SHAOYANG
CALM SPIRIT
SPASM VESSEL
BEN. EARS
CALM FRIGHT
& PACIFY WIND
YANG POND SOURCE
RELAX SINEWS & ALLEV. PAIN
REMOVE OBSTRUCT. CHAN.
CLEAR HEAT
PROMO. FLUID TRANS.
BEN. ORIGINAL QI
TON. CHONG & REN
BEN EARS
REG. SHAOYANG
HEAVENLY CREVICE
DISPEL W/D, REMOVE OBSTRUCT. CHAN.
UNBIND CHEST & REG. QI
CLEAR HEAT
BRANCH DITCH FIRE, RIVER, HORARY
REG. QI & BEN. CHEST & COSTAL REGION
REMOVE OBSTRUCT. CHAN.
CLEAR HEAT IN 3 JIAOS
EXPEL WIND
BEN. LI / MOVES STOOL
REG. REN
SHOULDER CREVICE
DISPEL W/D BI
ALLEV. PAIN / BEN. SHOULDER JOINT
OUTER PASS LUO, MASTER YANG WEI PT.
OPEN YANG WEI
EXPEL W/H & REL. EXT.
REMOVE OBSTRUCT.
BEN. EAR & HEAD
SUBDUE LV YANG
CLEAR HEAT IN HEAD
CONNECTING 3 YANG
CLEAR SJ CHANNEL
REMOVE OBSTRUCT. IN CHAN.
BEN. THROAT & VOICE
4 RIVERS
BEN. THROAT & EARS
CONVERGING CHANNELS XI-CLEFT
REMOVE OBSTRUCT. IN CHAN.
BEN. EARS
UPPER ARM MEETING
DISSIPATE NODULES
REG. QI & TRANS. PHLEGM
A.C.A.P.
DISPERSING RIVERBED
A.C.A.P.
CLEAR COLD ABYSS
ACTIVATE CHAN. & DISPEL W/D
CLEAR D/H
HEAVENLY WELL EARTH, HE-SEA, -SED.
CALM MIND
RESOLVE DAMP/PHLEGM (DISSIPATE NODULES)
CLEAR HEAT FROM SJ CHAN.
SUBDUE REBEL QI / REG. QI
1
2
3
4
5
6
7
8
9
10
11
12
13
14
15
16
17
18
19
20
21
22
23
SJ
SAN JIAO FXs

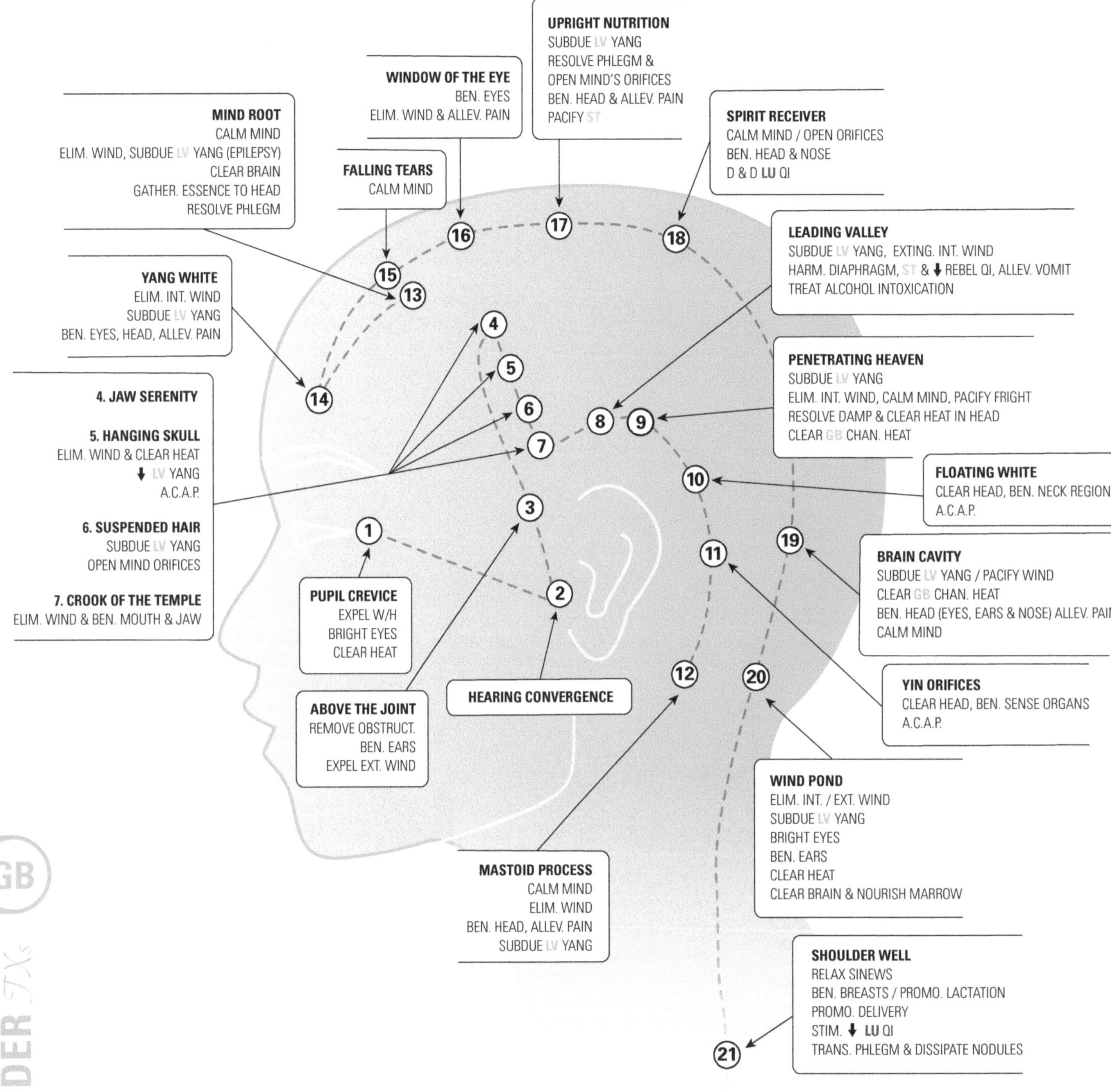
UPRIGHT NUTRITION
SUBDUE LV YANG
RESOLVE PHLEGM &
OPEN MIND'S ORIFICES
BEN. HEAD & ALLEV. PAIN
PACIFY ST
WINDOW OF THE EYE
BEN. EYES
ELIM. WIND & ALLEV. PAIN
MIND ROOT
CALM MIND
ELIM. WIND, SUBDUE LV YANG (EPILEPSY)
CLEAR BRAIN
GATHER. ESSENCE TO HEAD
RESOLVE PHLEGM
FALLING TEARS
CALM MIND
SPIRIT RECEIVER
CALM MIND / OPEN ORIFICES
BEN. HEAD & NOSE
D & D LU QI
LEADING VALLEY
SUBDUE LV YANG, EXTING. INT. WIND
HARM. DIAPHRAGM, ST & ↓ REBEL QI, ALLEV. VOMIT
TREAT ALCOHOL INTOXICATION
YANG WHITE
ELIM. INT. WIND
SUBDUE LV YANG
BEN. EYES, HEAD, ALLEV. PAIN
PENETRATING HEAVEN
SUBDUE LV YANG
ELIM. INT. WIND, CALM MIND, PACIFY FRIGHT
RESOLVE DAMP & CLEAR HEAT IN HEAD
CLEAR GB CHAN. HEAT
4. JAW SERENITY
5. HANGING SKULL
ELIM. WIND & CLEAR HEAT
↓ LV YANG
A.C.A.P.
6. SUSPENDED HAIR
SUBDUE LV YANG
OPEN MIND ORIFICES
7. CROOK OF THE TEMPLE
ELIM. WIND & BEN. MOUTH & JAW
FLOATING WHITE
CLEAR HEAD, BEN. NECK REGION
A.C.A.P.
BRAIN CAVITY
SUBDUE LV YANG / PACIFY WIND
CLEAR GB CHAN. HEAT
BEN. HEAD (EYES, EARS & NOSE) ALLEV. PAIN
CALM MIND
PUPIL CREVICE
EXPEL W/H
BRIGHT EYES
CLEAR HEAT
HEARING CONVERGENCE
ABOVE THE JOINT
REMOVE OBSTRUCT.
BEN. EARS
EXPEL EXT. WIND
YIN ORIFICES
CLEAR HEAD, BEN. SENSE ORGANS
A.C.A.P.
WIND POND
ELIM. INT. / EXT. WIND
SUBDUE LV YANG
BRIGHT EYES
BEN. EARS
CLEAR HEAT
CLEAR BRAIN & NOURISH MARROW
MASTOID PROCESS
CALM MIND
ELIM. WIND
BEN. HEAD, ALLEV. PAIN
SUBDUE LV YANG
SHOULDER WELL
RELAX SINEWS
BEN. BREASTS / PROMO. LACTATION
PROMO. DELIVERY
STIM. ↓ LU QI
TRANS. PHLEGM & DISSIPATE NODULES
1
2
3
4
5
6
7
8
9
10
11
12
13
14
15
16
17
18
19
20
21

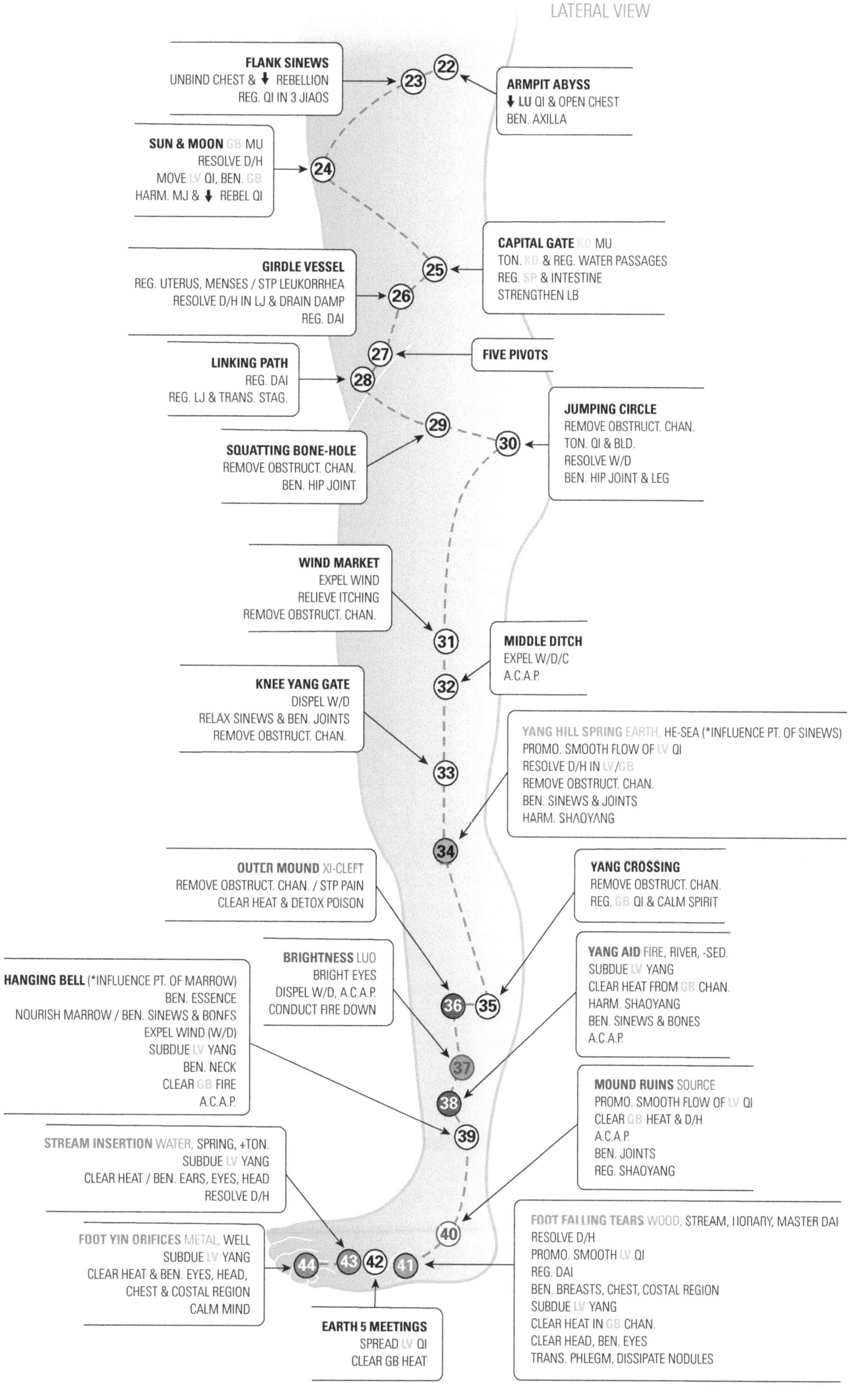

LATERAL VIEW
FLANK SINEWS
UNBIND CHEST & ↓ REBELLION
REG. QI IN 3 JIAOS
23
22
ARMPIT ABYSS
↓ LU QI & OPEN CHEST
BEN. AXILLA
SUN & MOON GB MU
RESOLVE D/H
MOVE LV QI, BEN. GB
HARM. MJ & ↓ REBEL QI
24
CAPITAL GATE KD MU
TON. KD & REG. WATER PASSAGES
REG. SP & INTESTINE
STRENGTHEN LB
25
GIRDLE VESSEL
REG. UTERUS, MENSES / STP LEUKORRHEA
RESOLVE D/H IN LJ & DRAIN DAMP
REG. DAI
26
27
FIVE PIVOTS
LINKING PATH
REG. DAI
REG. LJ & TRANS. STAG.
28
JUMPING CIRCLE
REMOVE OBSTRUCT. CHAN.
TON. QI & BLD.
RESOLVE W/D
BEN. HIP JOINT & LEG
29
30
SQUATTING BONE-HOLE
REMOVE OBSTRUCT. CHAN.
BEN. HIP JOINT
WIND MARKET
EXPEL WIND
RELIEVE ITCHING
REMOVE OBSTRUCT. CHAN.
31
MIDDLE DITCH
EXPEL W/D/C
A.C.A.P.
32
KNEE YANG GATE
DISPEL W/D
RELAX SINEWS & BEN. JOINTS
REMOVE OBSTRUCT. CHAN.
33
YANG HILL SPRING EARTH, HE-SEA (*INFLUENCE PT. OF SINEWS)
PROMO. SMOOTH FLOW OF LV QI
RESOLVE D/H IN LV/GB
REMOVE OBSTRUCT. CHAN.
BEN. SINEWS & JOINTS
HARM. SHAOYANG
34
OUTER MOUND XI-CLEFT
REMOVE OBSTRUCT. CHAN. / STP PAIN
CLEAR HEAT & DETOX POISON
YANG CROSSING
REMOVE OBSTRUCT. CHAN.
REG. GB QI & CALM SPIRIT
BRIGHTNESS LUO
BRIGHT EYES
DISPEL W/D, A.C.A.P.
CONDUCT FIRE DOWN
HANGING BELL (*INFLUENCE PT. OF MARROW)
BEN. ESSENCE
NOURISH MARROW / BEN. SINEWS & BONES
EXPEL WIND (W/D)
SUBDUE LV YANG
BEN. NECK
CLEAR GB FIRE
A.C.A.P.
36
35
YANG AID FIRE, RIVER, -SED.
SUBDUE LV YANG
CLEAR HEAT FROM GB CHAN.
HARM. SHAOYANG
BEN. SINEWS & BONES
A.C.A.P.
37
38
MOUND RUINS SOURCE
PROMO. SMOOTH FLOW OF LV QI
CLEAR GB HEAT & D/H
A.C.A.P.
BEN. JOINTS
REG. SHAOYANG
39
STREAM INSERTION WATER, SPRING, +TON.
SUBDUE LV YANG
CLEAR HEAT / BEN. EARS, EYES, HEAD
RESOLVE D/H
40
FOOT FALLING TEARS WOOD, STREAM, HORARY, MASTER DAI
RESOLVE D/H
PROMO. SMOOTH LV QI
REG. DAI
BEN. BREASTS, CHEST, COSTAL REGION
SUBDUE LV YANG
CLEAR HEAT IN GB CHAN.
CLEAR HEAD, BEN. EYES
TRANS. PHLEGM, DISSIPATE NODULES
FOOT YIN ORIFICES METAL, WELL
SUBDUE LV YANG
CLEAR HEAT & BEN. EYES, HEAD,
CHEST & COSTAL REGION
CALM MIND
44
43
42
41
EARTH 5 MEETINGS
SPREAD LV QI
CLEAR GB HEAT

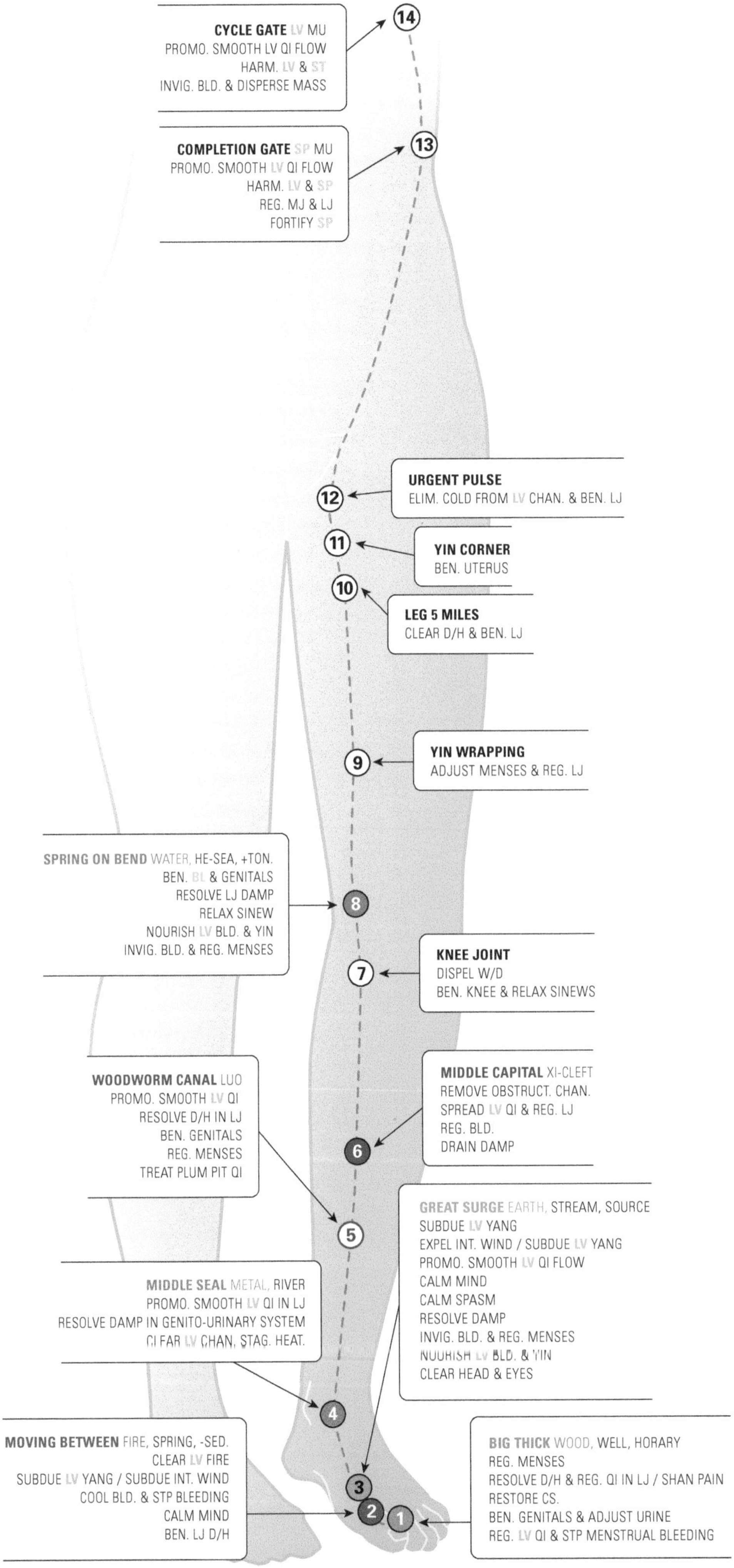

CYCLE GATE LV MU
PROMO. SMOOTH LV QI FLOW
HARM. LV & ST
INVIG. BLD. & DISPERSE MASS

14

COMPLETION GATE SP MU
PROMO. SMOOTH LV QI FLOW
HARM. LV & SP
REG. MJ & LJ
FORTIFY SP

13

URGENT PULSE
ELIM. COLD FROM LV CHAN. & BEN. LJ

12

11

YIN CORNER
BEN. UTERUS

10

LEG 5 MILES
CLEAR D/H & BEN. LJ

YIN WRAPPING
ADJUST MENSES & REG. LJ

9

SPRING ON BEND WATER, HE-SEA, +TON.
BEN. BL & GENITALS
RESOLVE LJ DAMP
RELAX SINEW
NOURISH LV BLD. & YIN
INVIG. BLD. & REG. MENSES

8

KNEE JOINT
DISPEL W/D
BEN. KNEE & RELAX SINEWS

7

MIDDLE CAPITAL XI-CLEFT
REMOVE OBSTRUCT. CHAN.
SPREAD LV QI & REG. LJ
REG. BLD.
DRAIN DAMP

6

WOODWORM CANAL LUO
PROMO. SMOOTH LV QI
RESOLVE D/H IN LJ
BEN. GENITALS
REG. MENSES
TREAT PLUM PIT QI

5

GREAT SURGE EARTH, STREAM, SOURCE
SUBDUE LV YANG
EXPEL INT. WIND / SUBDUE LV YANG
PROMO. SMOOTH LV QI FLOW
CALM MIND
CALM SPASM
RESOLVE DAMP
INVIG. BLD. & REG. MENSES
NOURISH LV BLD. & YIN
CLEAR HEAD & EYES

MIDDLE SEAL METAL, RIVER
PROMO. SMOOTH LV QI IN LJ
RESOLVE DAMP IN GENITO-URINARY SYSTEM
CLEAR LV CHAN. STAG. HEAT.

4

MOVING BETWEEN FIRE, SPRING, -SED.
CLEAR LV FIRE
SUBDUE LV YANG / SUBDUE INT. WIND
COOL BLD. & STP BLEEDING
CALM MIND
BEN. LJ D/H

3

2

1

BIG THICK WOOD, WELL, HORARY
REG. MENSES
RESOLVE D/H & REG. QI IN LJ / SHAN PAIN
RESTORE CS.
BEN. GENITALS & ADJUST URINE
REG. LV QI & STP MENSTRUAL BLEEDING

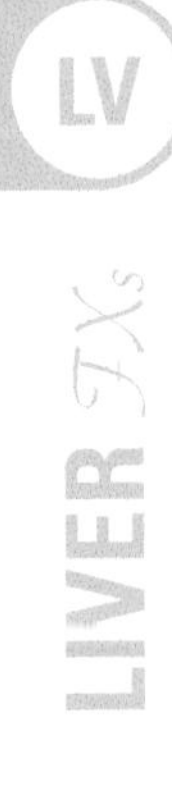

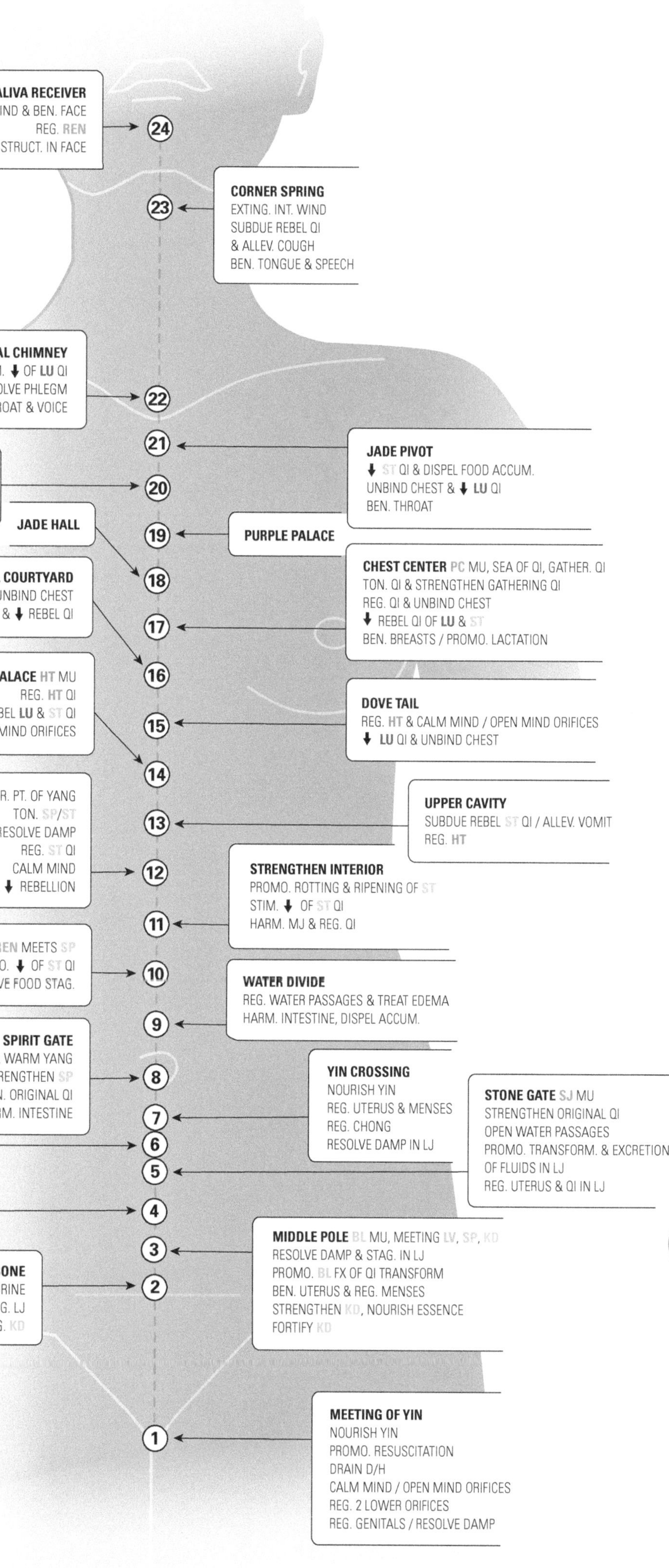

SALIVA RECEIVER → 24
EXTING. INT. WIND & BEN. FACE
REG. REN
REMOVE OBSTRUCT. IN FACE

CORNER SPRING → 23
EXTING. INT. WIND
SUBDUE REBEL QI
& ALLEV. COUGH
BEN. TONGUE & SPEECH

CELESTIAL CHIMNEY → 22
STIM. ⬇ OF **LU** QI
RESOLVE PHLEGM
BEN. THROAT & VOICE

JADE PIVOT → 21
⬇ ST QI & DISPEL FOOD ACCUM.
UNBIND CHEST & ⬇ **LU** QI
BEN. THROAT

MAGNIFICENT CANOPY → 20
UNBIND CHEST
REG. & ⬇ QI

PURPLE PALACE → 19

JADE HALL → 18

CHEST CENTER PC MU, SEA OF QI, GATHER. QI → 17
TON. QI & STRENGTHEN GATHERING QI
REG. QI & UNBIND CHEST
⬇ REBEL QI OF **LU** & ST
BEN. BREASTS / PROMO. LACTATION

CENTRAL COURTYARD → 16
UNBIND CHEST
REG. ST & ⬇ REBEL QI

DOVE TAIL → 15
REG. **HT** & CALM MIND / OPEN MIND ORIFICES
⬇ **LU** QI & UNBIND CHEST

GREAT PALACE HT MU → 14
REG. **HT** QI
SUBDUE REBEL **LU** & ST QI
CALM MIND, TRANS. PHLEGM / OPEN MIND ORIFICES

UPPER CAVITY → 13
SUBDUE REBEL ST QI / ALLEV. VOMIT
REG. **HT**

MIDDLE CAVITY ST MU, GATHER. PT. OF YANG → 12
TON. SP/ST
RESOLVE DAMP
REG. ST QI
CALM MIND
HARM. MJ & ⬇ REBELLION

STRENGTHEN INTERIOR → 11
PROMO. ROTTING & RIPENING OF ST
STIM. ⬇ OF ST QI
HARM. MJ & REG. QI

LOWER CAVITY REN MEETS SP → 10
PROMO. ⬇ OF ST QI
RELIEVE FOOD STAG.

WATER DIVIDE → 9
REG. WATER PASSAGES & TREAT EDEMA
HARM. INTESTINE, DISPEL ACCUM.

SPIRIT GATE → 8
RESCUE & WARM YANG
STRENGTHEN SP
TON. ORIGINAL QI
WARM & HARM. INTESTINE

YIN CROSSING → 7
NOURISH YIN
REG. UTERUS & MENSES
REG. CHONG
RESOLVE DAMP IN LJ

SEA OF QI → 6
TON. QI & YANG
RAISE SINKING QI, RESCUE COLLAPSE OF YANG
TON. ORIGINAL QI
REG. QI IN LJ & HARM. BLD.
TON. KD & FORTIFY YANG

STONE GATE SJ MU → 5
STRENGTHEN ORIGINAL QI
OPEN WATER PASSAGES
PROMO. TRANSFORM. & EXCRETION
OF FLUIDS IN LJ
REG. UTERUS & QI IN LJ

GATE TO THE ORIGINAL QI SI MU → 4
NOURISH BLD. & YIN
STRENGTHEN UTERUS & REG. MENSES
BEN. ORIGINAL QI, BEN. ESSENCE
STRENGTHEN KD
ROOTS SHEN & HUN, RESTORE COLLAPSE
BEN. BL, REG. **SI** / REG. LJ
WARM & FORTIFY SP

MIDDLE POLE BL MU, MEETING LV, SP, KD → 3
RESOLVE DAMP & STAG. IN LJ
PROMO. BL FX OF QI TRANSFORM
BEN. UTERUS & REG. MENSES
STRENGTHEN KD, NOURISH ESSENCE
FORTIFY KD

CURVED BONE → 2
BEN. URINE
REG. LJ
WARM & INVIG. KD

MEETING OF YIN → 1
NOURISH YIN
PROMO. RESUSCITATION
DRAIN D/H
CALM MIND / OPEN MIND ORIFICES
REG. 2 LOWER ORIFICES
REG. GENITALS / RESOLVE DAMP

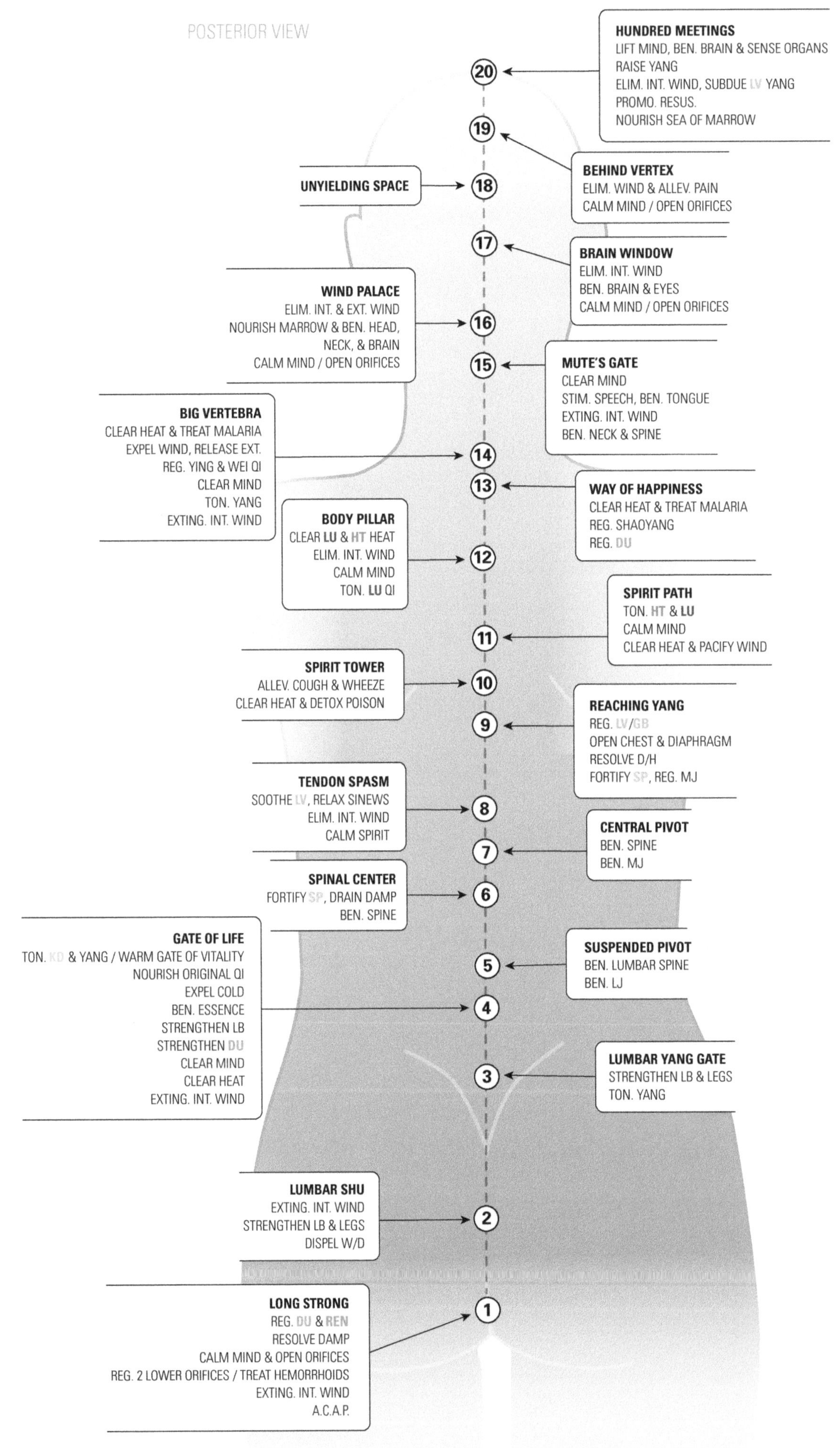

POSTERIOR VIEW
HUNDRED MEETINGS
LIFT MIND, BEN. BRAIN & SENSE ORGANS
RAISE YANG
ELIM. INT. WIND, SUBDUE LV YANG
PROMO. RESUS.
NOURISH SEA OF MARROW
20
19
BEHIND VERTEX
ELIM. WIND & ALLEV. PAIN
CALM MIND / OPEN ORIFICES
UNYIELDING SPACE
18
17
BRAIN WINDOW
ELIM. INT. WIND
BEN. BRAIN & EYES
CALM MIND / OPEN ORIFICES
WIND PALACE
ELIM. INT. & EXT. WIND
NOURISH MARROW & BEN. HEAD, NECK, & BRAIN
CALM MIND / OPEN ORIFICES
16
15
MUTE'S GATE
CLEAR MIND
STIM. SPEECH, BEN. TONGUE
EXTING. INT. WIND
BEN. NECK & SPINE
BIG VERTEBRA
CLEAR HEAT & TREAT MALARIA
EXPEL WIND, RELEASE EXT.
REG. YING & WEI QI
CLEAR MIND
TON. YANG
EXTING. INT. WIND
14
13
WAY OF HAPPINESS
CLEAR HEAT & TREAT MALARIA
REG. SHAOYANG
REG. DU
BODY PILLAR
CLEAR LU & HT HEAT
ELIM. INT. WIND
CALM MIND
TON. LU QI
12
SPIRIT PATH
TON. HT & LU
CALM MIND
CLEAR HEAT & PACIFY WIND
11
SPIRIT TOWER
ALLEV. COUGH & WHEEZE
CLEAR HEAT & DETOX POISON
10
9
REACHING YANG
REG. LV/GB
OPEN CHEST & DIAPHRAGM
RESOLVE D/H
FORTIFY SP, REG. MJ
TENDON SPASM
SOOTHE LV, RELAX SINEWS
ELIM. INT. WIND
CALM SPIRIT
8
7
CENTRAL PIVOT
BEN. SPINE
BEN. MJ
SPINAL CENTER
FORTIFY SP, DRAIN DAMP
BEN. SPINE
6
GATE OF LIFE
TON. KD & YANG / WARM GATE OF VITALITY
NOURISH ORIGINAL QI
EXPEL COLD
BEN. ESSENCE
STRENGTHEN LB
STRENGTHEN DU
CLEAR MIND
CLEAR HEAT
EXTING. INT. WIND
5
SUSPENDED PIVOT
BEN. LUMBAR SPINE
BEN. LJ
4
3
LUMBAR YANG GATE
STRENGTHEN LB & LEGS
TON. YANG
LUMBAR SHU
EXTING. INT. WIND
STRENGTHEN LB & LEGS
DISPEL W/D
2
LONG STRONG
REG. DU & REN
RESOLVE DAMP
CALM MIND & OPEN ORIFICES
REG. 2 LOWER ORIFICES / TREAT HEMORRHOIDS
EXTING. INT. WIND
A.C.A.P.
1

IN FRONT OF THE CROWN (21)
ELIM. WIND & TREAT CONVULSIONS
BEN. HEAD

FONTANELLE MEETING (22)
BEN. NOSE
ELIM. WIND & BEN. HEAD

MIND COURTYARD (23)
CALM & LIFT MIND, OPEN MIND ORIFICES, BEN. BRAIN
BEN. NOSE & EYES
EXTING. INT. WIND & BEN. HEAD

UPPER STAR (24)
OPEN NOSE, BEN. EYES
ELIM. WIND, BEN. HEAD & FACE, & DISPEL SWELL
CALM SPIRIT

WHITE CREVICE (25)
BEN. NOSE

MAN'S MIDDLE (26)
PROMO. RESUS. & EXTING. INT. WIND
CALM MIND & OPEN MIND ORIFICES
BEN. LUMBAR SPINE & TREAT ACUTE LUMBAR SPRAIN
OPEN NOSE
REG. UJ WATER PASSAGES

EXTREMITY OF MOUTH (27)
CLEAR HEAT, GENERATE FLUIDS, & BEN. MOUTH
CALM SPIRIT

GUM INTERSECTION (28)
CLEAR HEAT & BEN. GUMS
BEN. NOSE & EYES

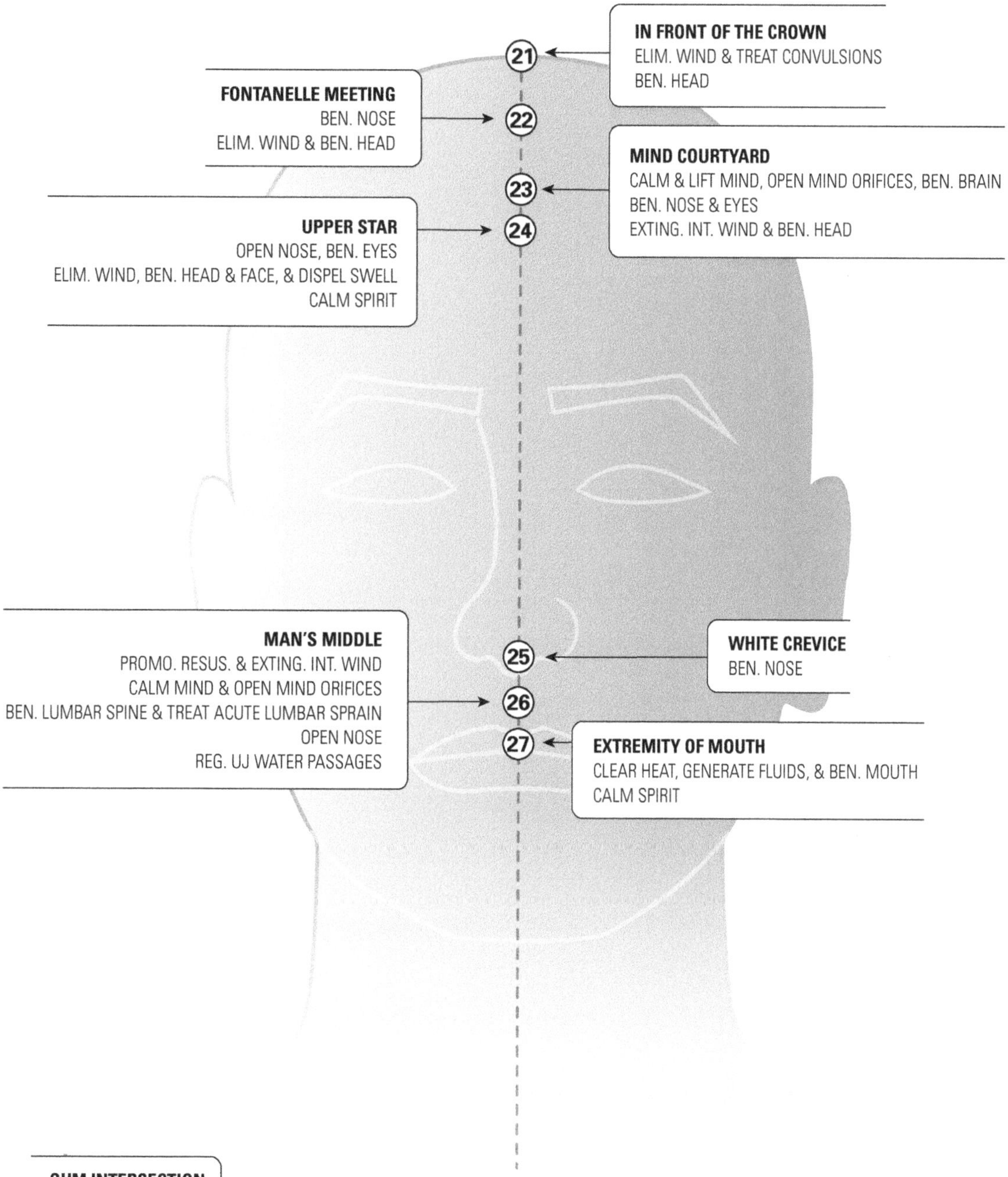

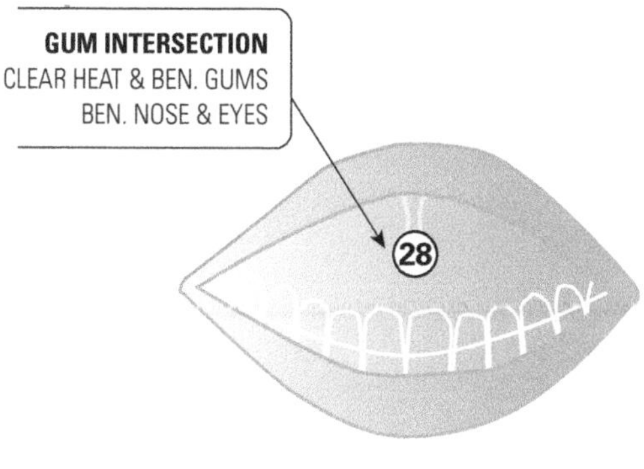

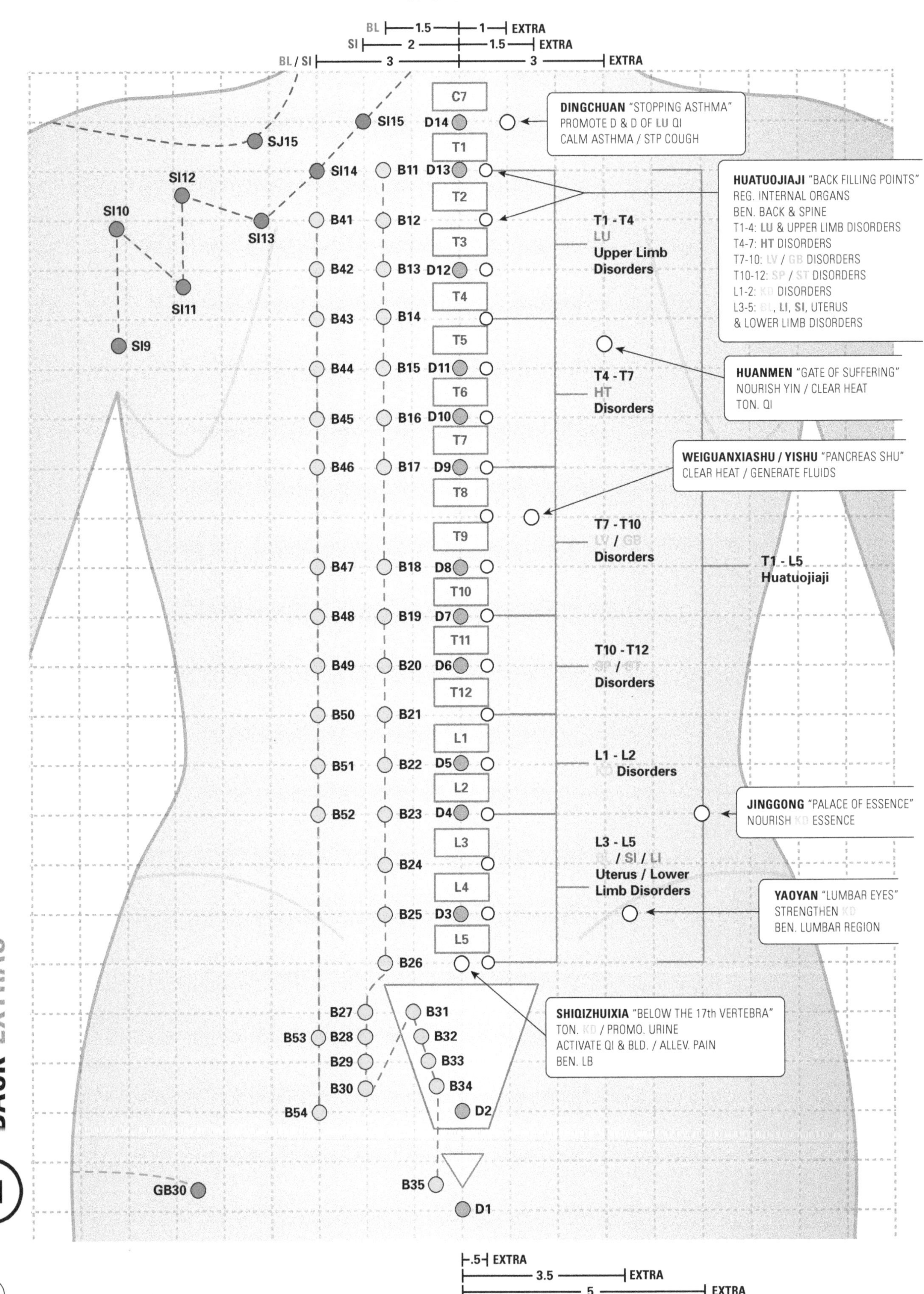
POSTERIOR VIEW
BL 1.5 1 EXTRA
SI 2 1.5 EXTRA
BL / SI 3 3 EXTRA
C7 T1 T2 T3 T4 T5 T6 T7 T8 T9 T10 T11 T12 L1 L2 L3 L4 L5
SI15 D14 SJ15 SI14 B11 D13 SI12 SI10 B41 B12 SI13 B42 B13 D12 SI11 B43 B14 SI9 B44 B15 D11 B45 B16 D10 B46 B17 D9 B47 B18 D8 B48 B19 D7 B49 B20 D6 B50 B21 B51 B22 D5 B52 B23 D4 B24 B25 D3 B26 B27 B31 B53 B28 B32 B29 B33 B30 B34 B54 D2 B35 GB30 D1
DINGCHUAN "STOPPING ASTHMA"
PROMOTE D & D OF LU QI
CALM ASTHMA / STP COUGH
HUATUOJIAJI "BACK FILLING POINTS"
REG. INTERNAL ORGANS
BEN. BACK & SPINE
T1-4: LU & UPPER LIMB DISORDERS
T4-7: HT DISORDERS
T7-10: LV / GB DISORDERS
T10-12: SP / ST DISORDERS
L1-2: KD DISORDERS
L3-5: BL, LI, SI, UTERUS
& LOWER LIMB DISORDERS
T1 - T4
LU
Upper Limb
Disorders
HUANMEN "GATE OF SUFFERING"
NOURISH YIN / CLEAR HEAT
TON. QI
T4 - T7
HT
Disorders
WEIGUANXIASHU / YISHU "PANCREAS SHU"
CLEAR HEAT / GENERATE FLUIDS
T7 - T10
LV / GB
Disorders
T1 - L5
Huatuojiaji
T10 - T12
SP / ST
Disorders
L1 - L2
KD Disorders
JINGGONG "PALACE OF ESSENCE"
NOURISH KD ESSENCE
L3 - L5
BL / SI / LI
Uterus / Lower
Limb Disorders
YAOYAN "LUMBAR EYES"
STRENGTHEN KD
BEN. LUMBAR REGION
SHIQIZHUIXIA "BELOW THE 17th VERTEBRA"
TON. KD / PROMO. URINE
ACTIVATE QI & BLD. / ALLEV. PAIN
BEN. LB
.5 EXTRA
3.5 EXTRA
5 EXTRA

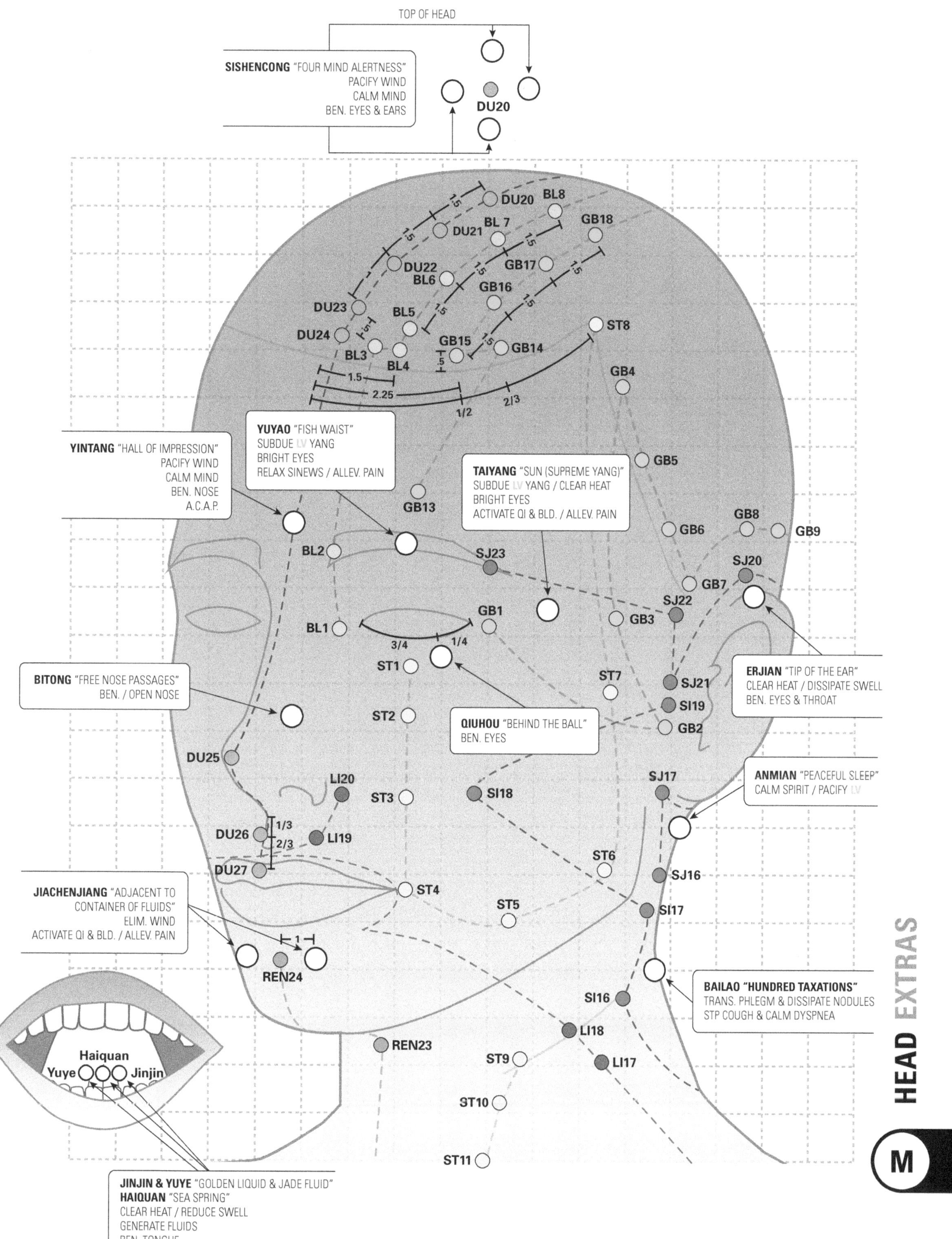

HEAD EXTRAS

M

ANTERIOR VIEW

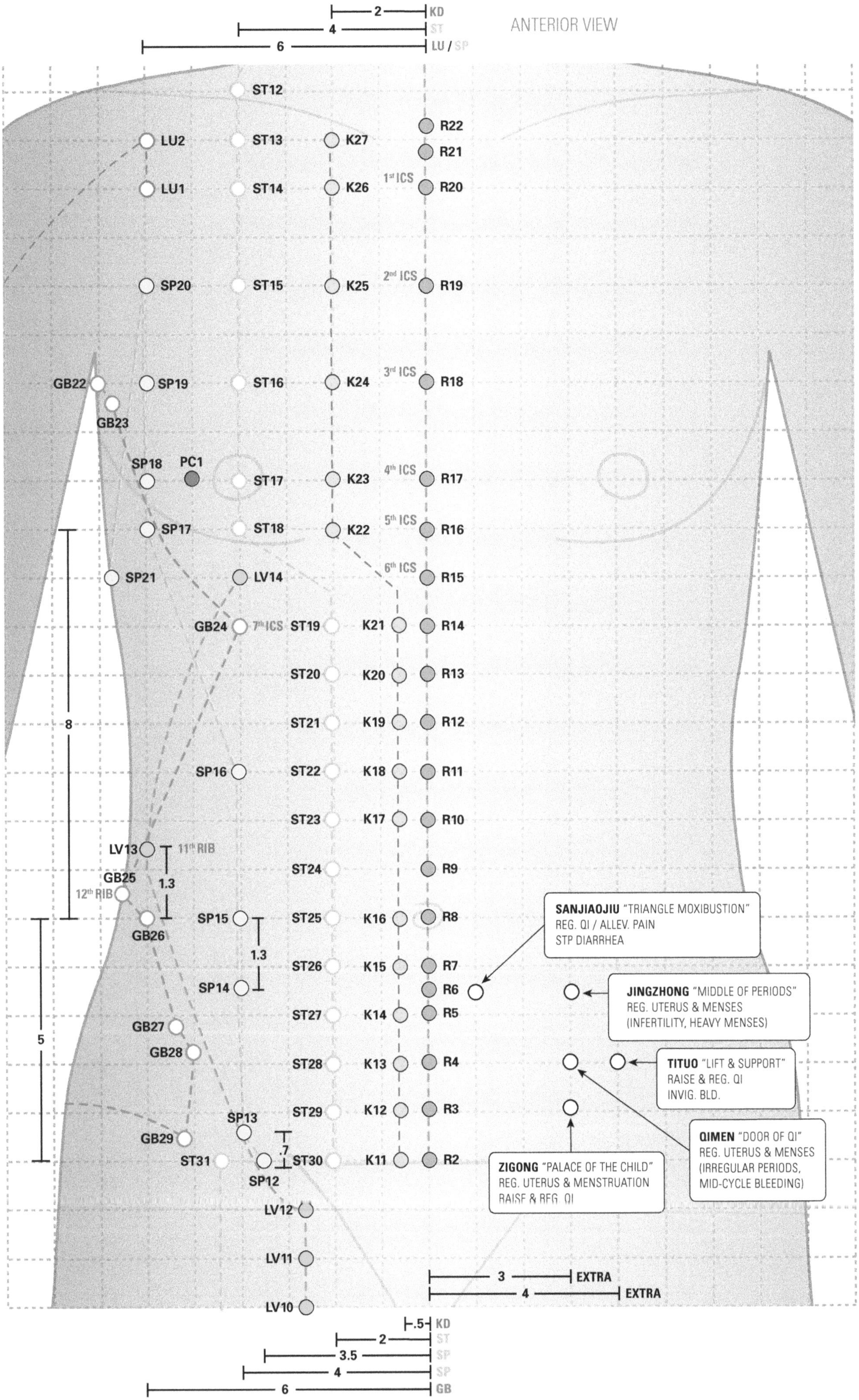

2 KD
4 ST
6 LU / SP

ST12
LU2 ST13 K27 R22
R21
LU1 ST14 K26 1st ICS R20
SP20 ST15 K25 2nd ICS R19
GB22 SP19 ST16 K24 3rd ICS R18
GB23
SP18 PC1 ST17 K23 4th ICS R17
SP17 ST18 K22 5th ICS R16
SP21 LV14 6th ICS R15
GB24 7th ICS ST19 K21 R14
ST20 K20 R13
8
ST21 K19 R12
SP16 ST22 K18 R11
ST23 K17 R10
LV13 11th RIB
GB25 1.3 ST24 R9
12th RIB
GB26 SP15 ST25 K16 R8
1.3
ST26 K15 R7
SP14 R6
ST27 K14 R5
5
GB27
GB28 ST28 K13 R4
SP13 ST29 K12 R3
GB29 .7
ST31 SP12 ST30 K11 R2
LV12
LV11
LV10

SANJIAOJIU "TRIANGLE MOXIBUSTION"
REG. QI / ALLEV. PAIN
STP DIARRHEA

JINGZHONG "MIDDLE OF PERIODS"
REG. UTERUS & MENSES
(INFERTILITY, HEAVY MENSES)

TITUO "LIFT & SUPPORT"
RAISE & REG. QI
INVIG. BLD.

QIMEN "DOOR OF QI"
REG. UTERUS & MENSES
(IRREGULAR PERIODS, MID-CYCLE BLEEDING)

ZIGONG "PALACE OF THE CHILD"
REG. UTERUS & MENSTRUATION
RAISE & REG. QI

3 EXTRA
4 EXTRA

.5 KD
2 ST
3.5 SP
4 SP
6 GB

TORSO EXTRAS

M

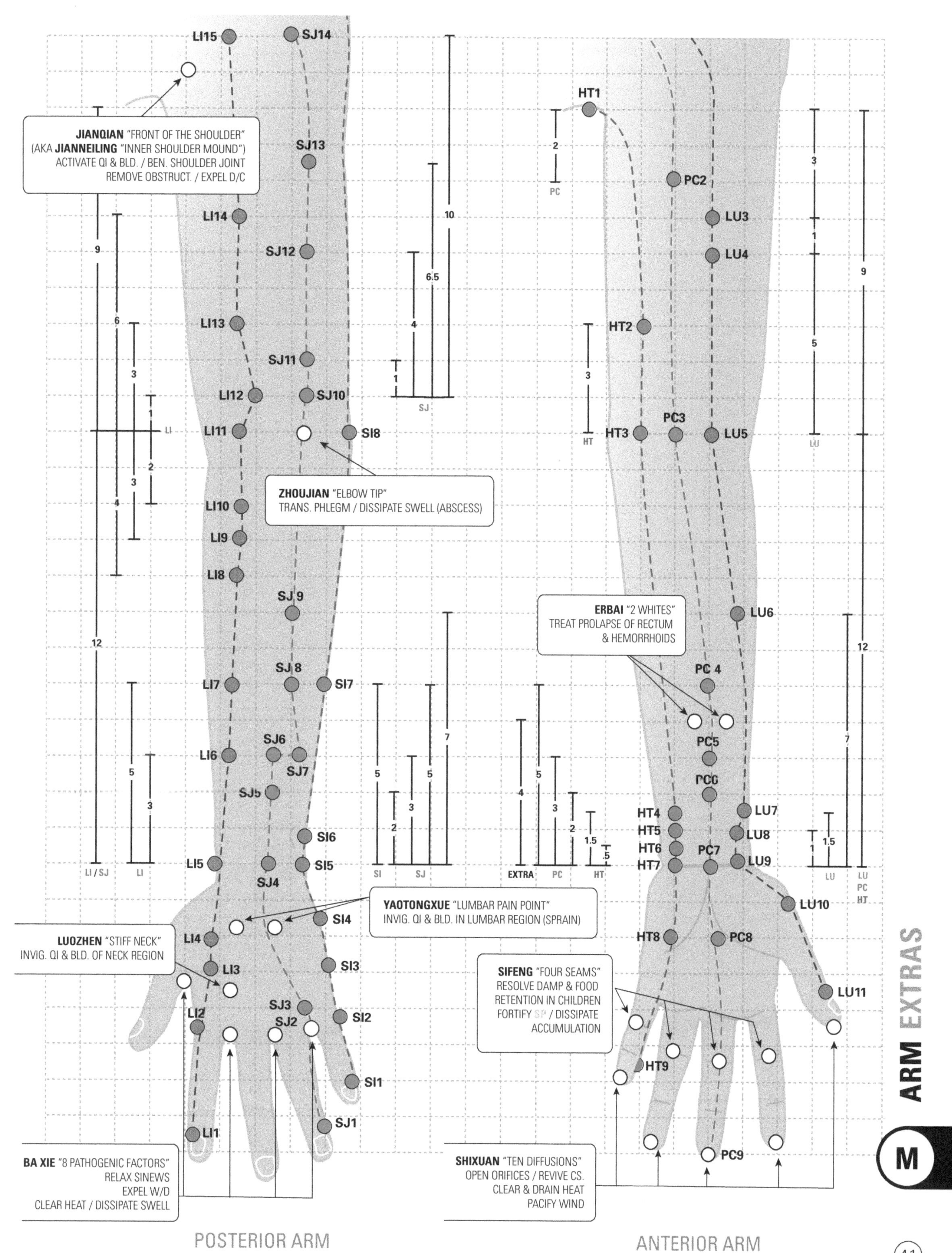
JIANQIAN "FRONT OF THE SHOULDER"
(AKA JIANNEILING "INNER SHOULDER MOUND")
ACTIVATE QI & BLD. / BEN. SHOULDER JOINT
REMOVE OBSTRUCT. / EXPEL D/C
ZHOUJIAN "ELBOW TIP"
TRANS. PHLEGM / DISSIPATE SWELL (ABSCESS)
YAOTONGXUE "LUMBAR PAIN POINT"
INVIG. QI & BLD. IN LUMBAR REGION (SPRAIN)
LUOZHEN "STIFF NECK"
INVIG. QI & BLD. OF NECK REGION
BA XIE "8 PATHOGENIC FACTORS"
RELAX SINEWS
EXPEL W/D
CLEAR HEAT / DISSIPATE SWELL
ERBAI "2 WHITES"
TREAT PROLAPSE OF RECTUM
& HEMORRHOIDS
SIFENG "FOUR SEAMS"
RESOLVE DAMP & FOOD
RETENTION IN CHILDREN
FORTIFY SP / DISSIPATE
ACCUMULATION
SHIXUAN "TEN DIFFUSIONS"
OPEN ORIFICES / REVIVE CS.
CLEAR & DRAIN HEAT
PACIFY WIND
LI15 SJ14 SJ13 LI14 SJ12 LI13 SJ11 LI12 SJ10 LI11 SI8 LI10 LI9 LI8 SJ 9 SJ 8 LI7 SI7 SJ6 LI6 SJ7 SJ5 SI6 LI5 SI5 SJ4 SI4 LI4 LI3 SI3 LI2 SJ3 SJ2 SI2 SI1 LI1 SJ1
HT1 PC2 LU3 LU4 HT2 PC3 HT3 LU5 LU6 PC 4 PC5 PC6 HT4 LU7 HT5 LU8 HT6 PC7 HT7 LU9 LU10 HT8 PC8 LU11 HT9 PC9
LI / SJ
LI
SJ
SI
EXTRA
PC
HT
LU
LU PC HT
POSTERIOR ARM
ANTERIOR ARM
ARM EXTRAS
M

LEG EXTRAS

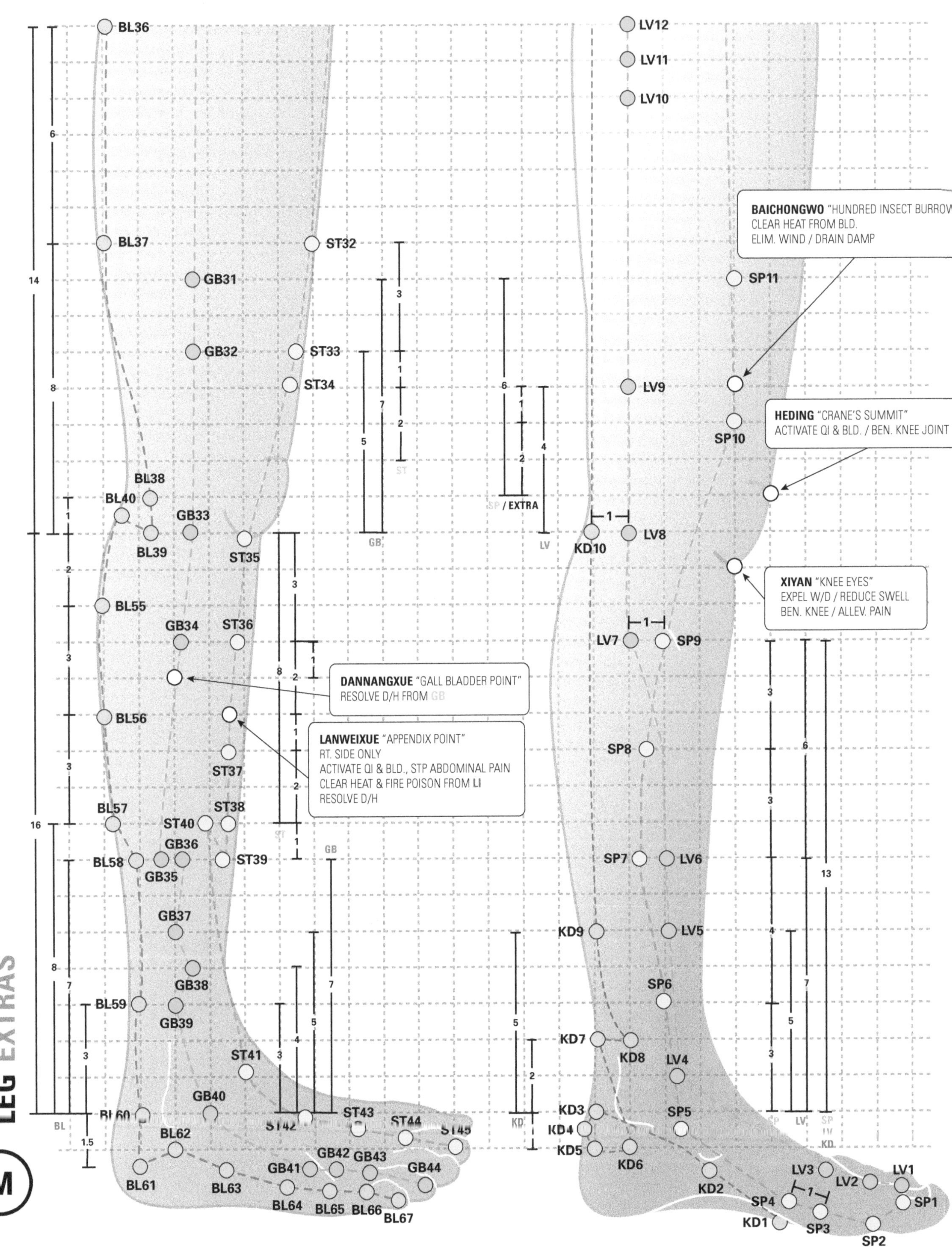

LATERAL POSTERIOR

MEDIAL ANTERIOR

Part 2

The Acupuncture Point Functions Charts Workbook

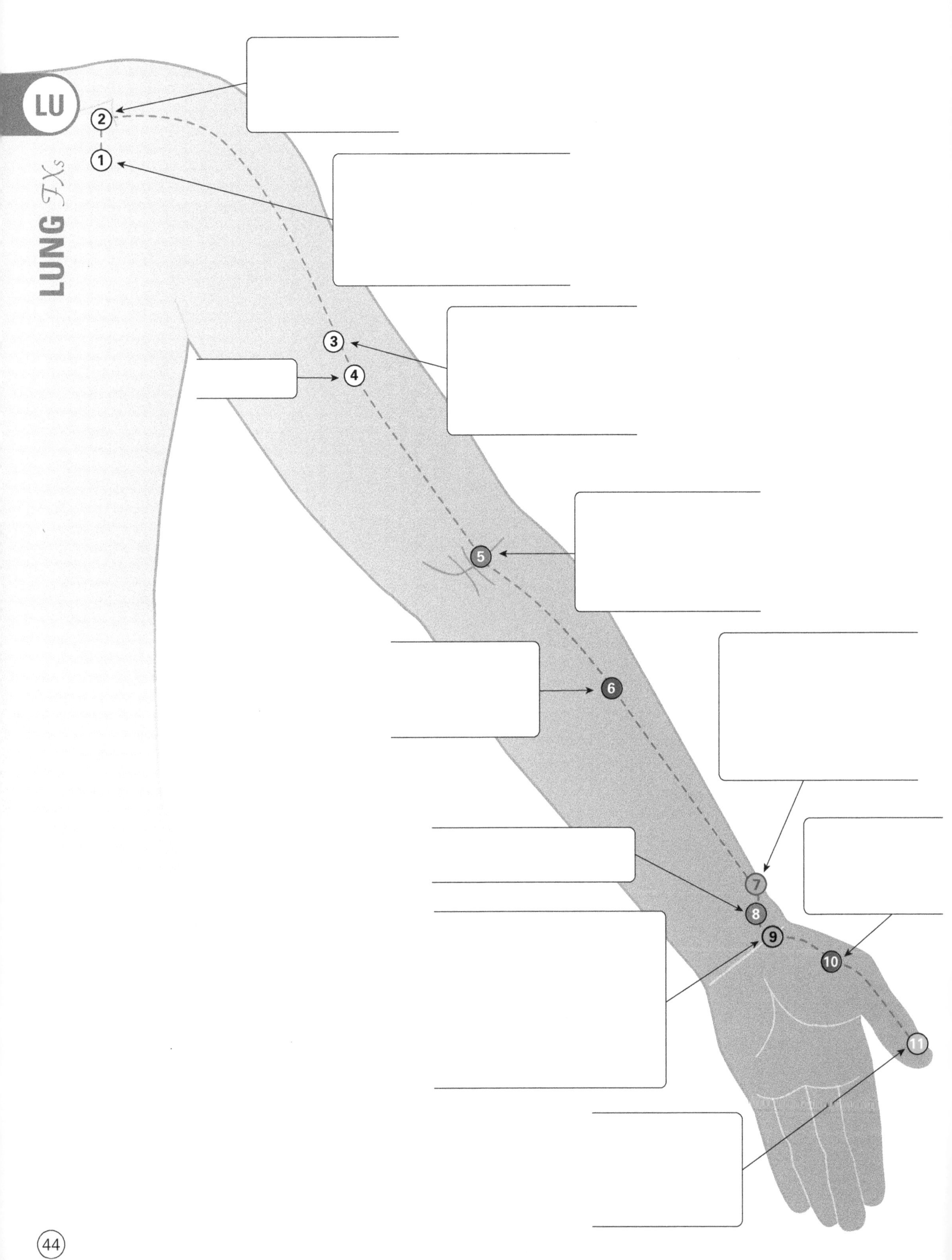
LU
LUNG FXs
2
1
3
4
5
6
7
8
9
10
11

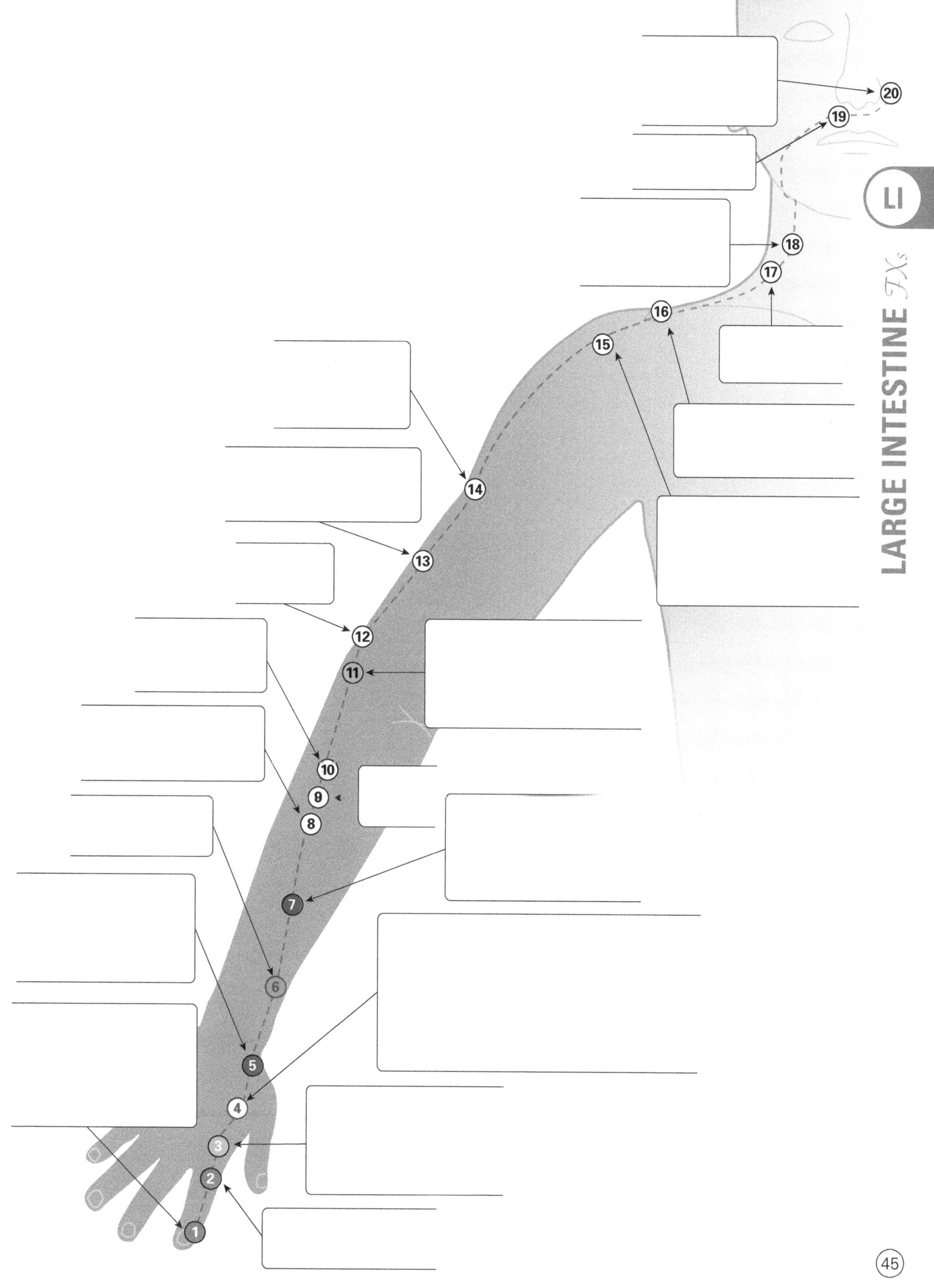

LI
LARGE INTESTINE FXs
20
19
18
17
16
15
14
13
12
11
10
9
8
7
6
5
4
3
2
1

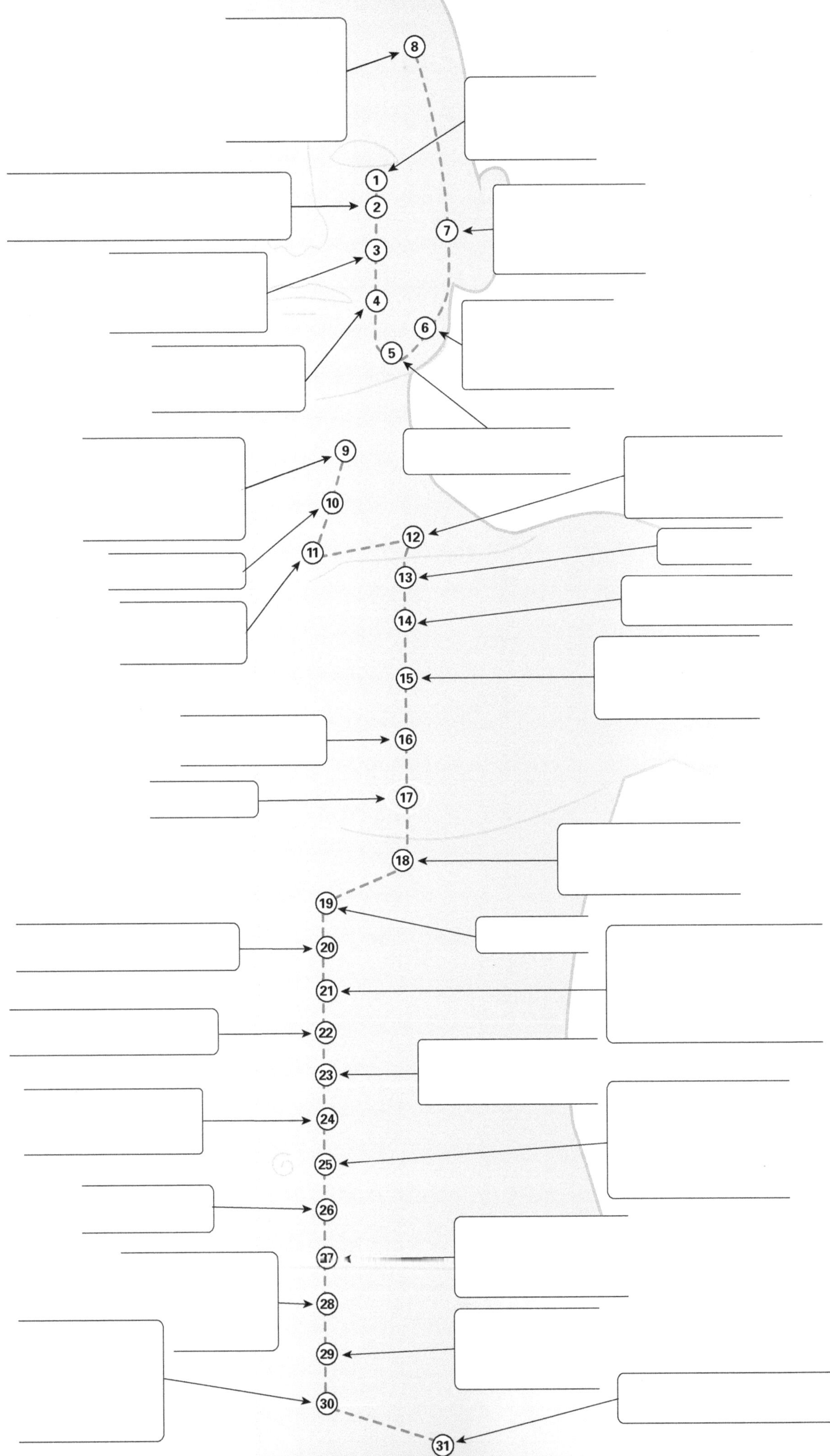
8
1
2
7
3
4
6
5
9
10
12
11
13
14
15
16
17
18
19
20
21
22
23
24
25
26
27
28
29
30
31

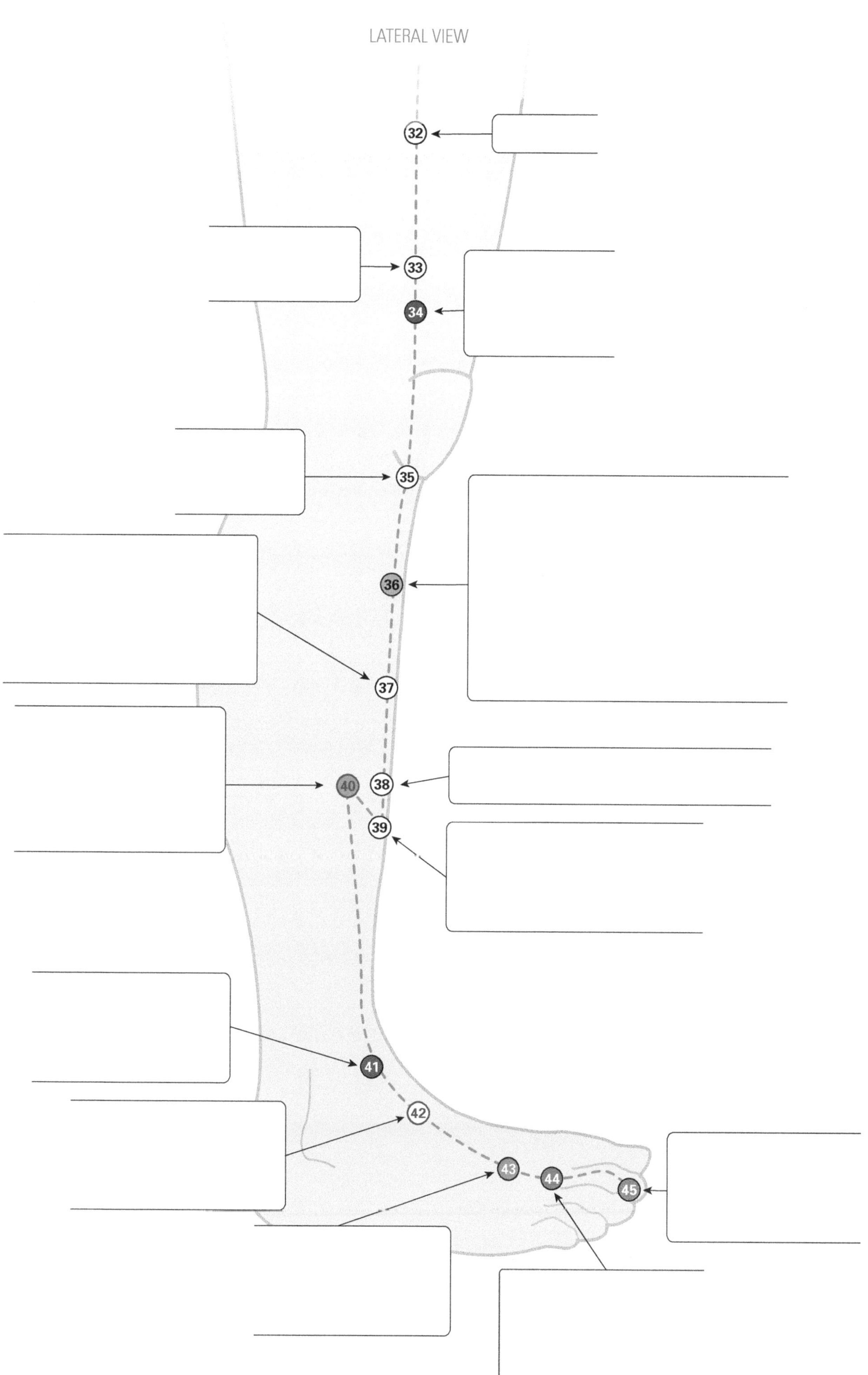
LATERAL VIEW
32
33
34
35
36
37
38
39
40
41
42
43
44
45

SPLEEN FXs

SP

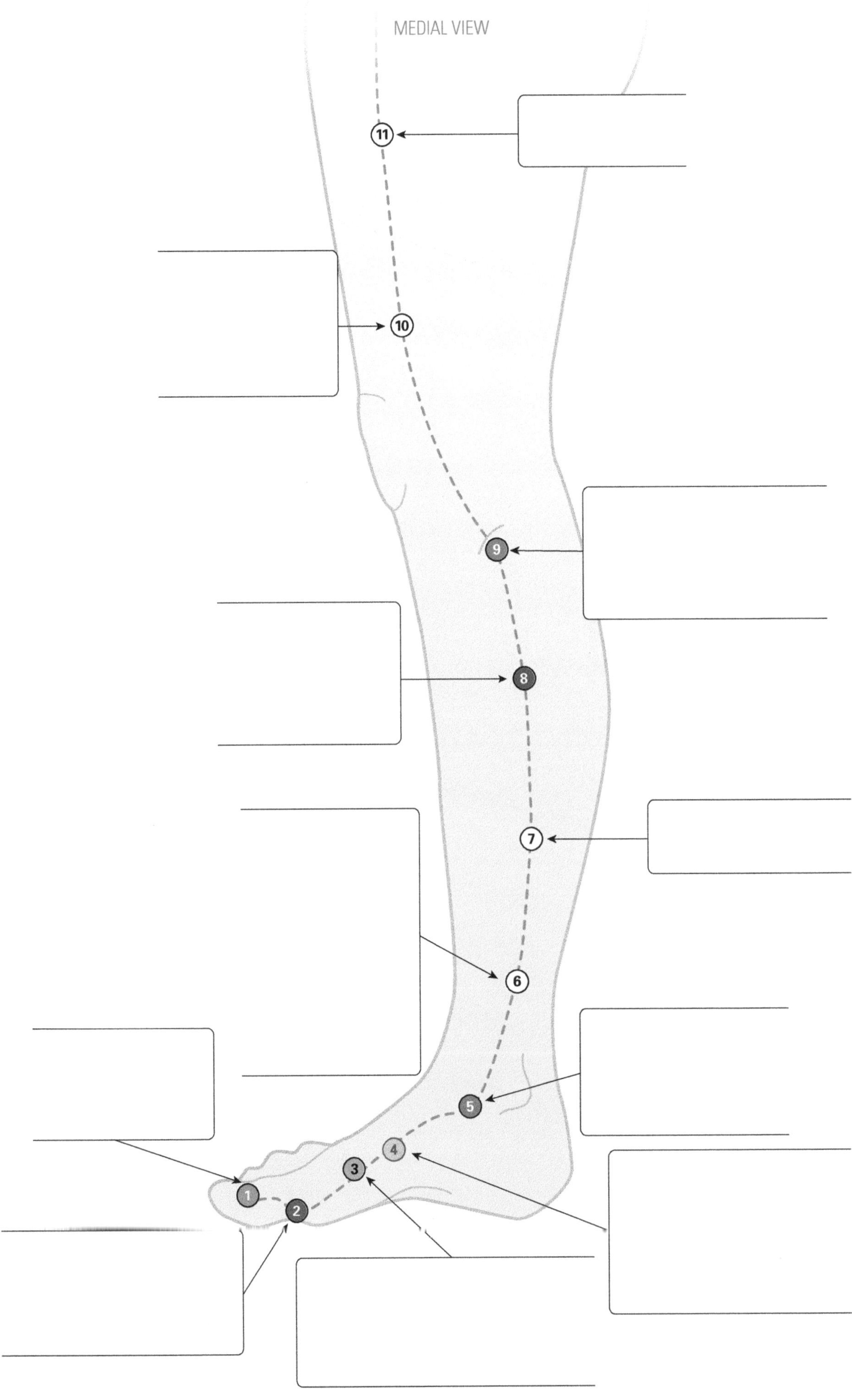

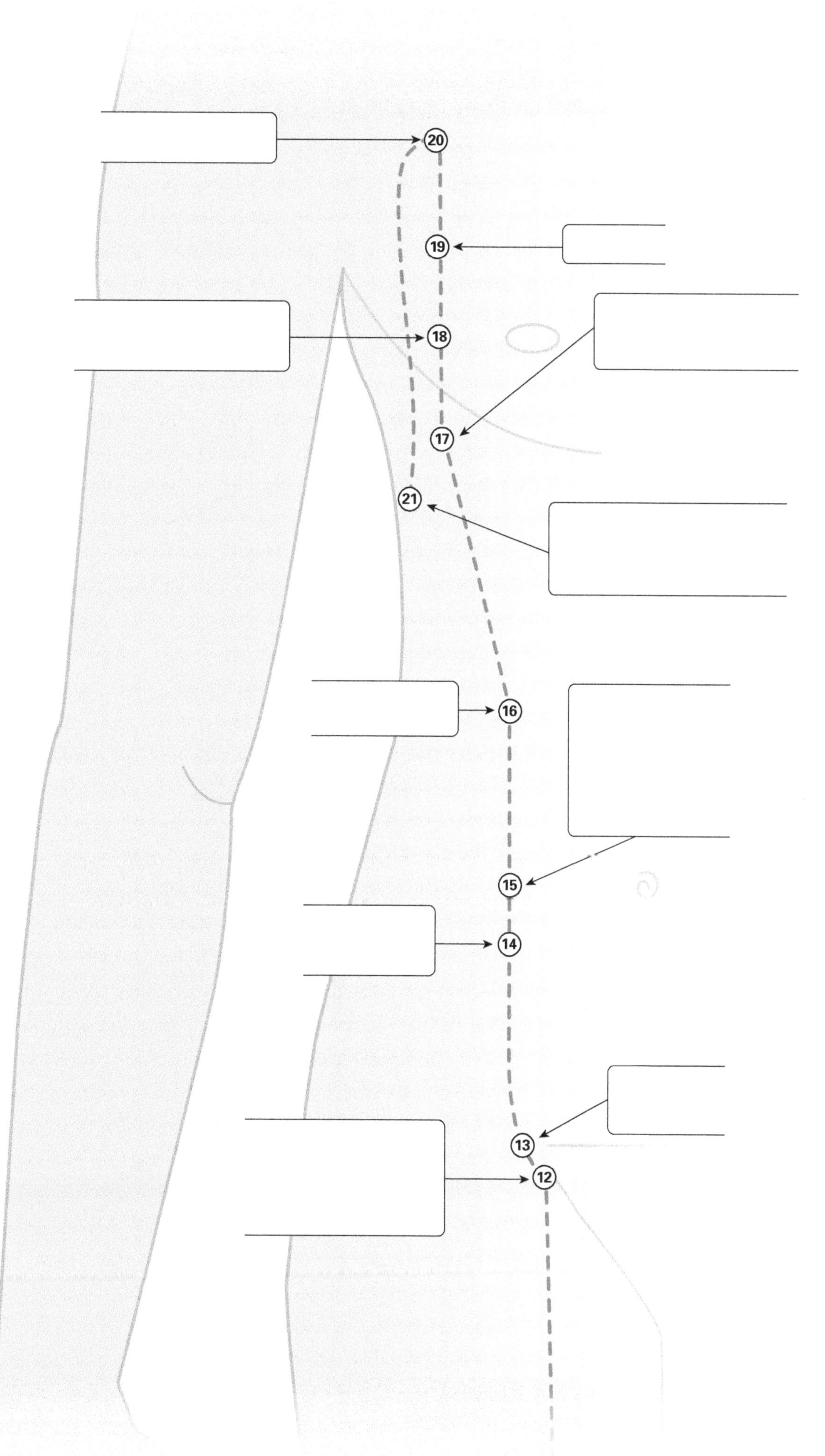
20
19
18
17
21
16
15
14
13
12

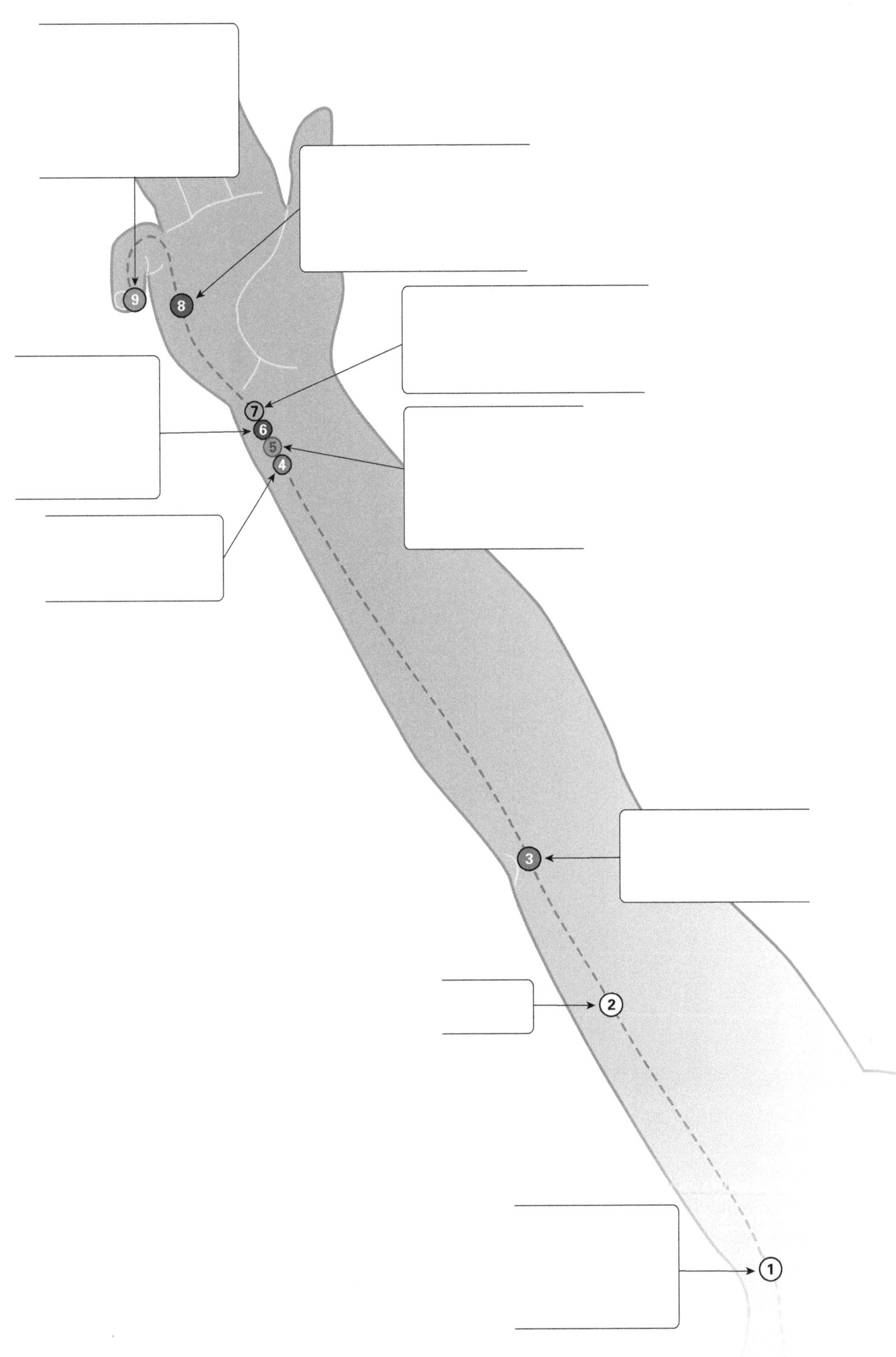
9
8
7
6
5
4
3
2
1

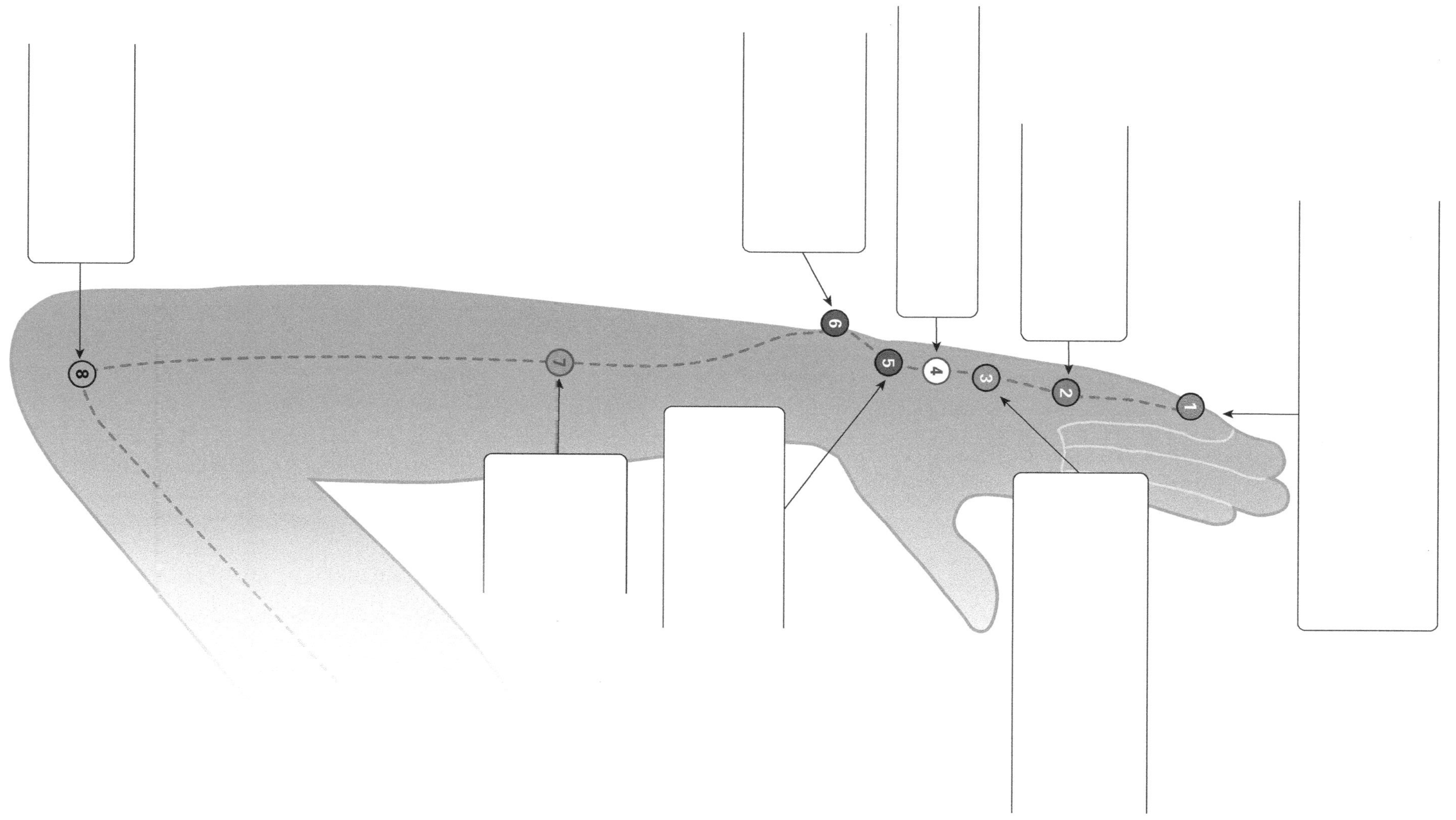
8
7
6
5
4
3
2
1

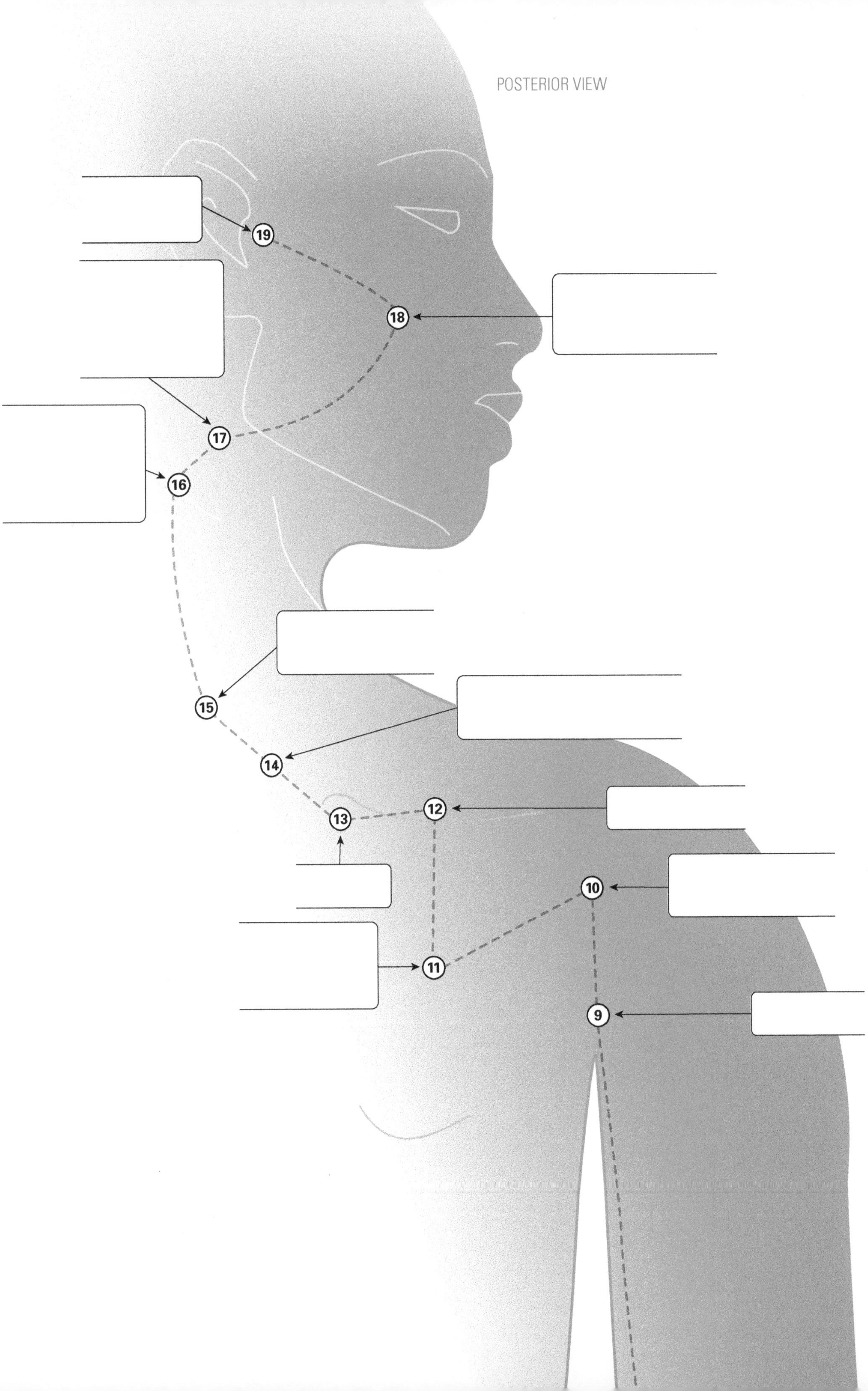

POSTERIOR VIEW

19

18

17

16

15

14

12

13

10

11

9

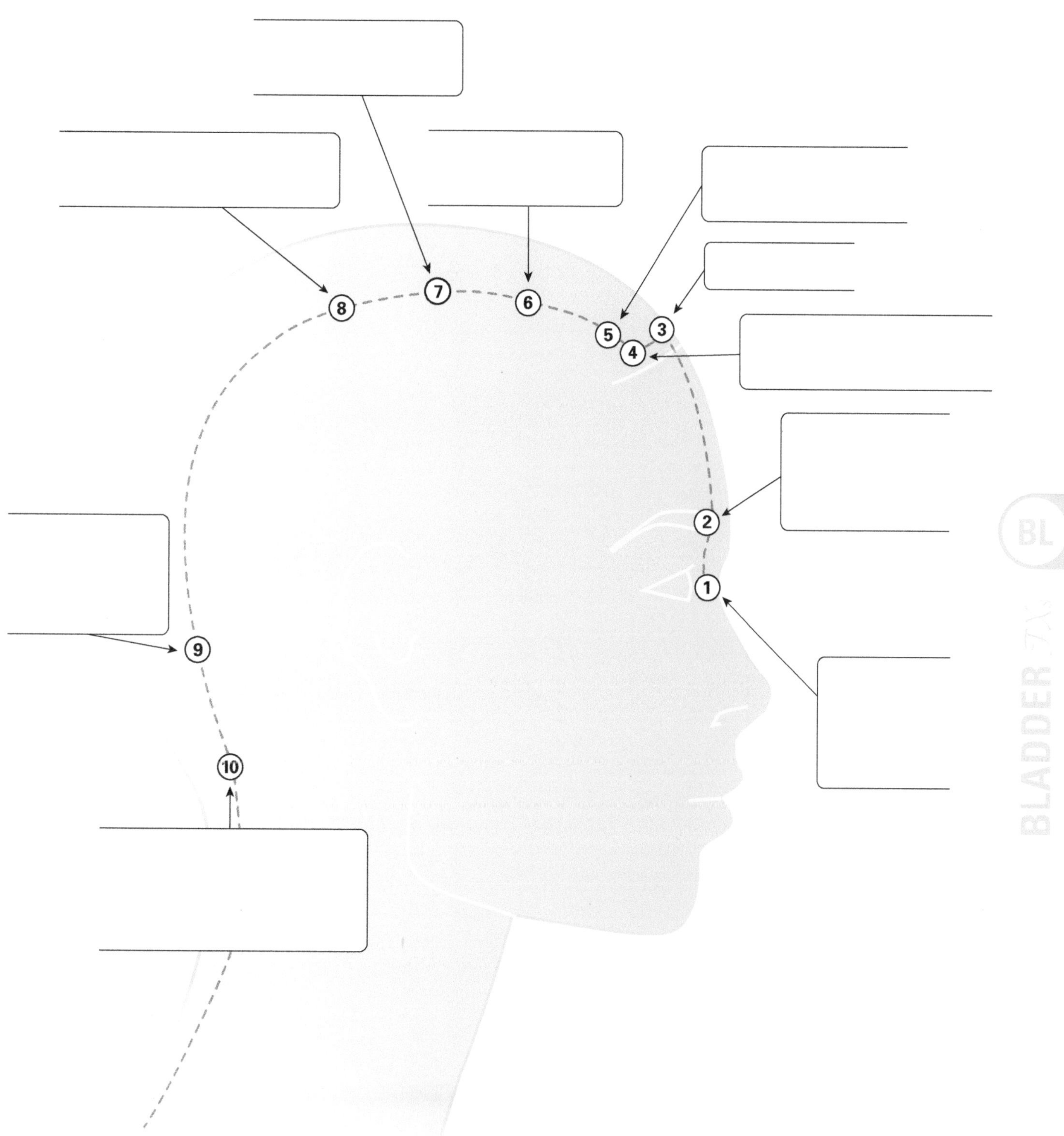
1
2
3
4
5
6
7
8
9
10

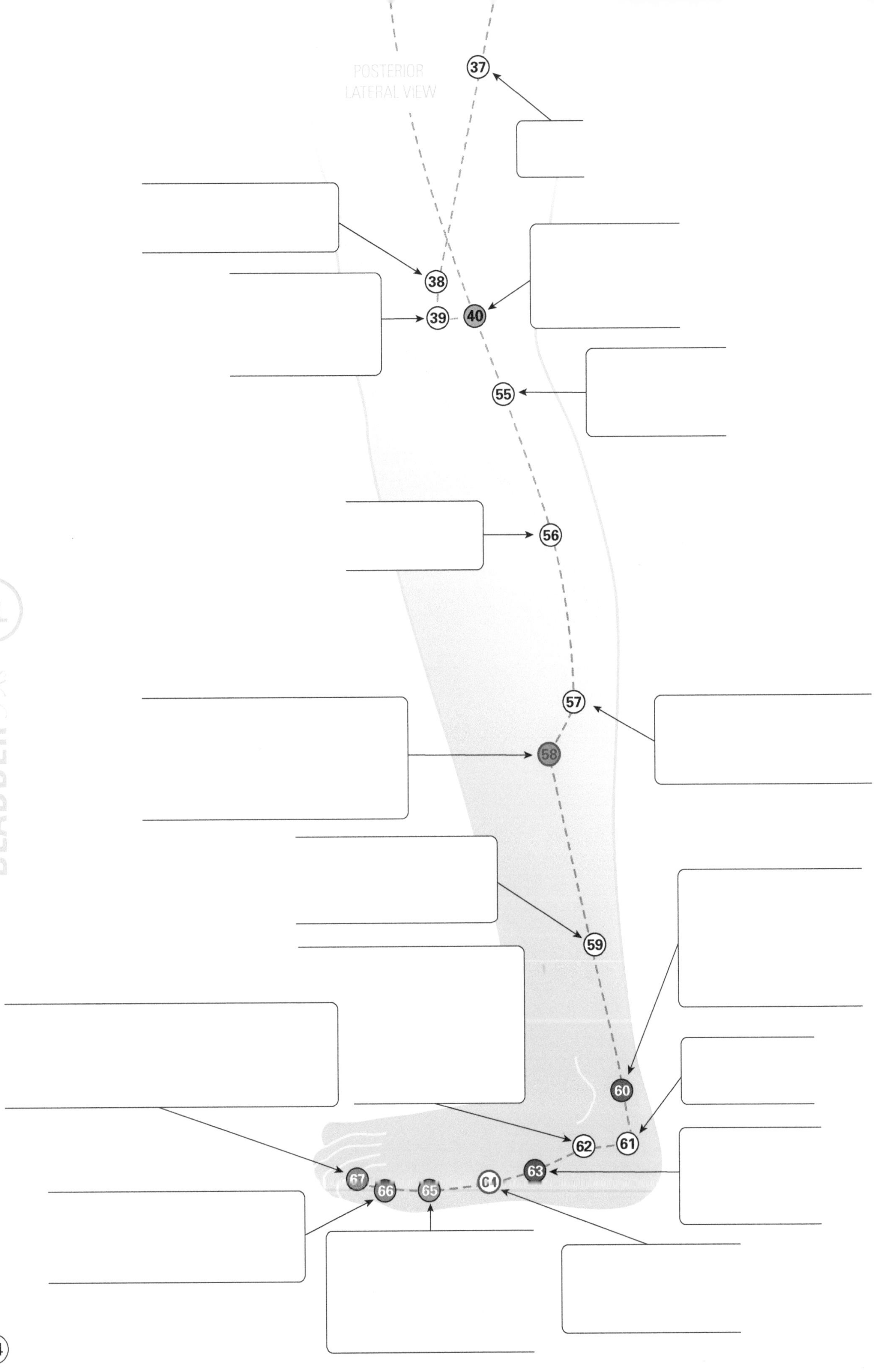

POSTERIOR LATERAL VIEW

37

38

39

40

55

56

57

58

59

60

61

62

63

64

65

66

67

BL

BLADDER

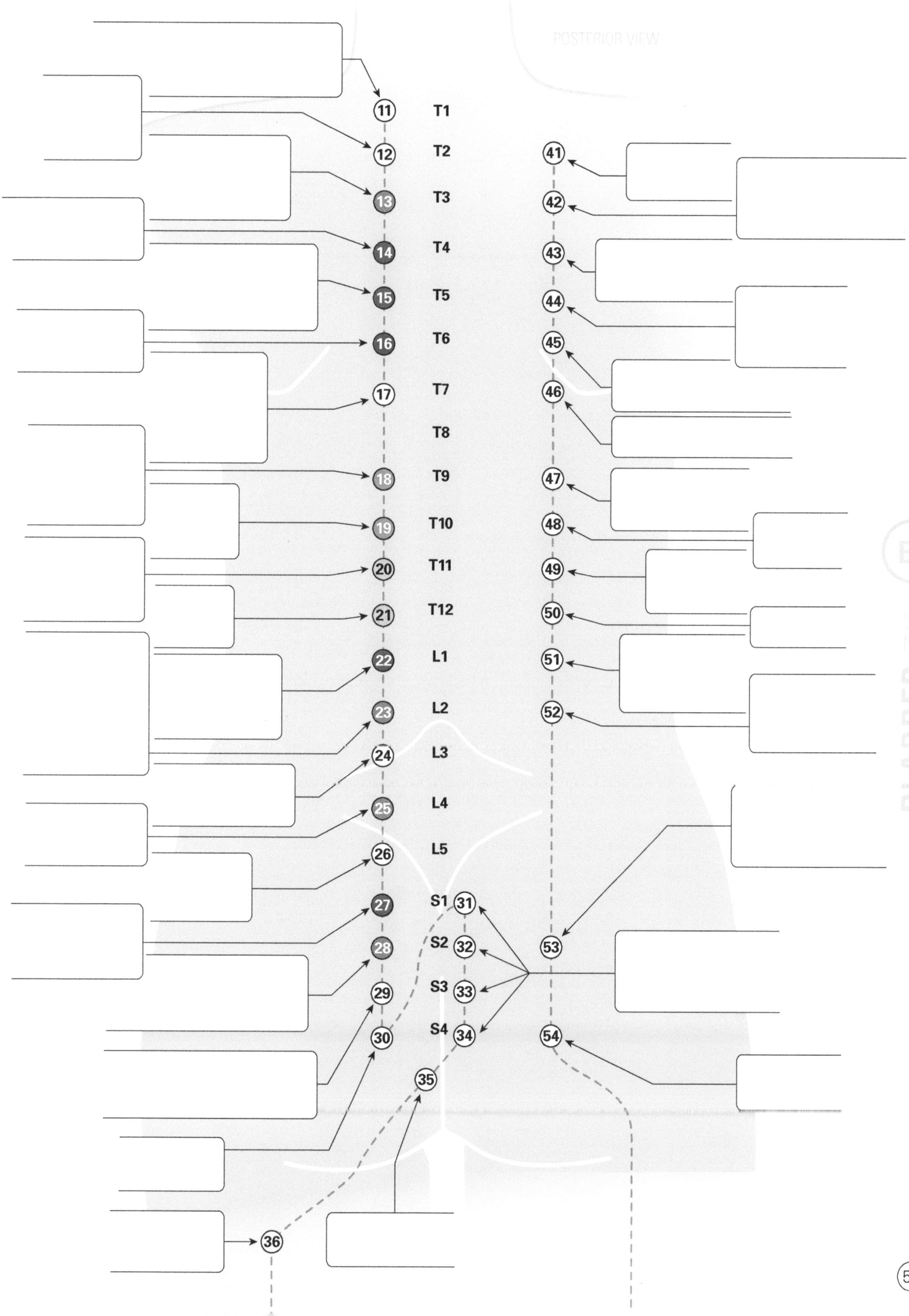

POSTERIOR VIEW

11 T1
12 T2 41
13 T3 42
14 T4 43
15 T5 44
16 T6 45
17 T7 46
T8
18 T9 47
19 T10 48
20 T11 49
21 T12 50
22 L1 51
23 L2 52
24 L3
25 L4
26 L5
27 S1 31
28 S2 32 53
29 S3 33
30 S4 34 54
35
36

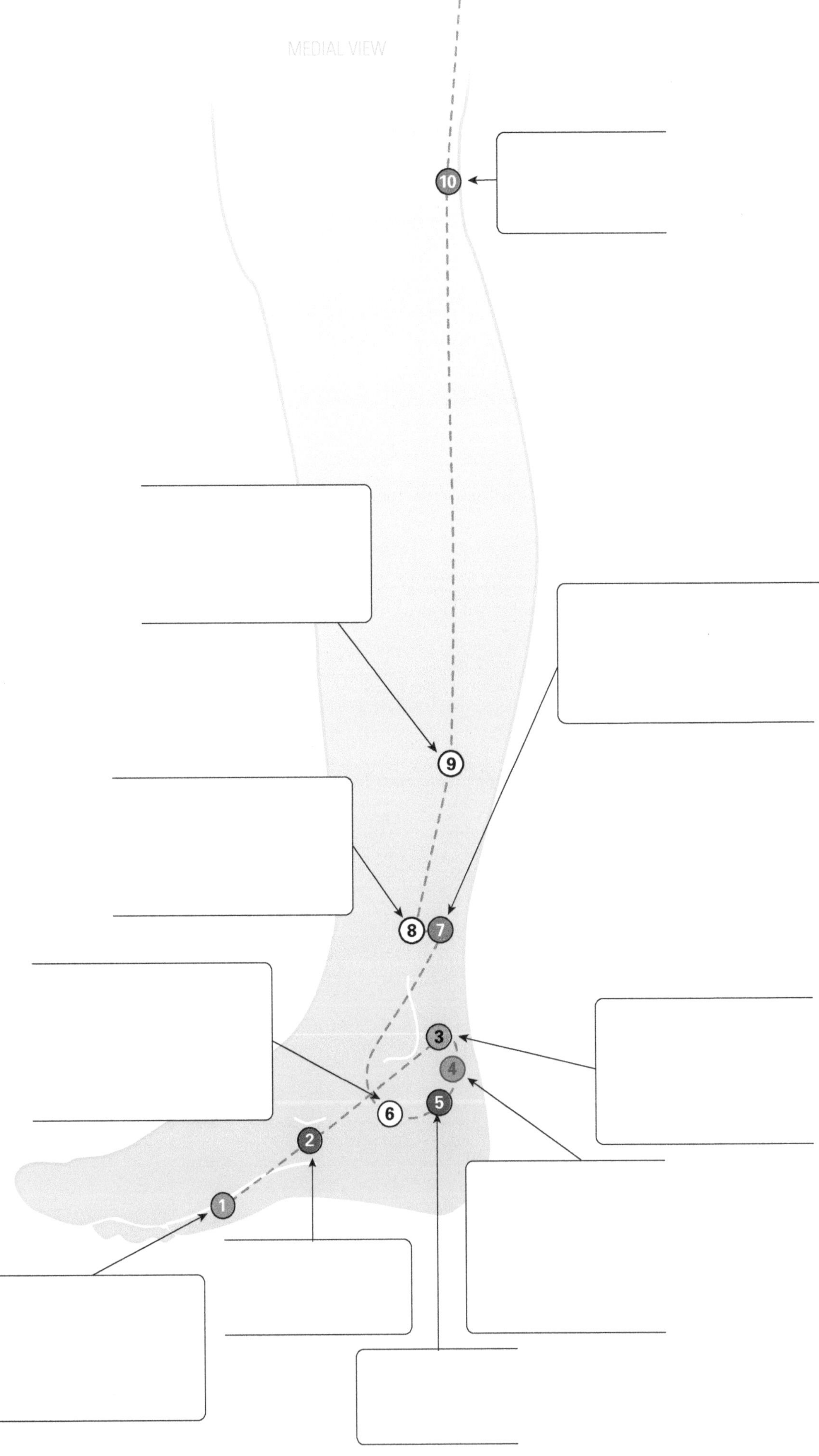
MEDIAL VIEW
10
9
8
7
3
4
6
5
2
1

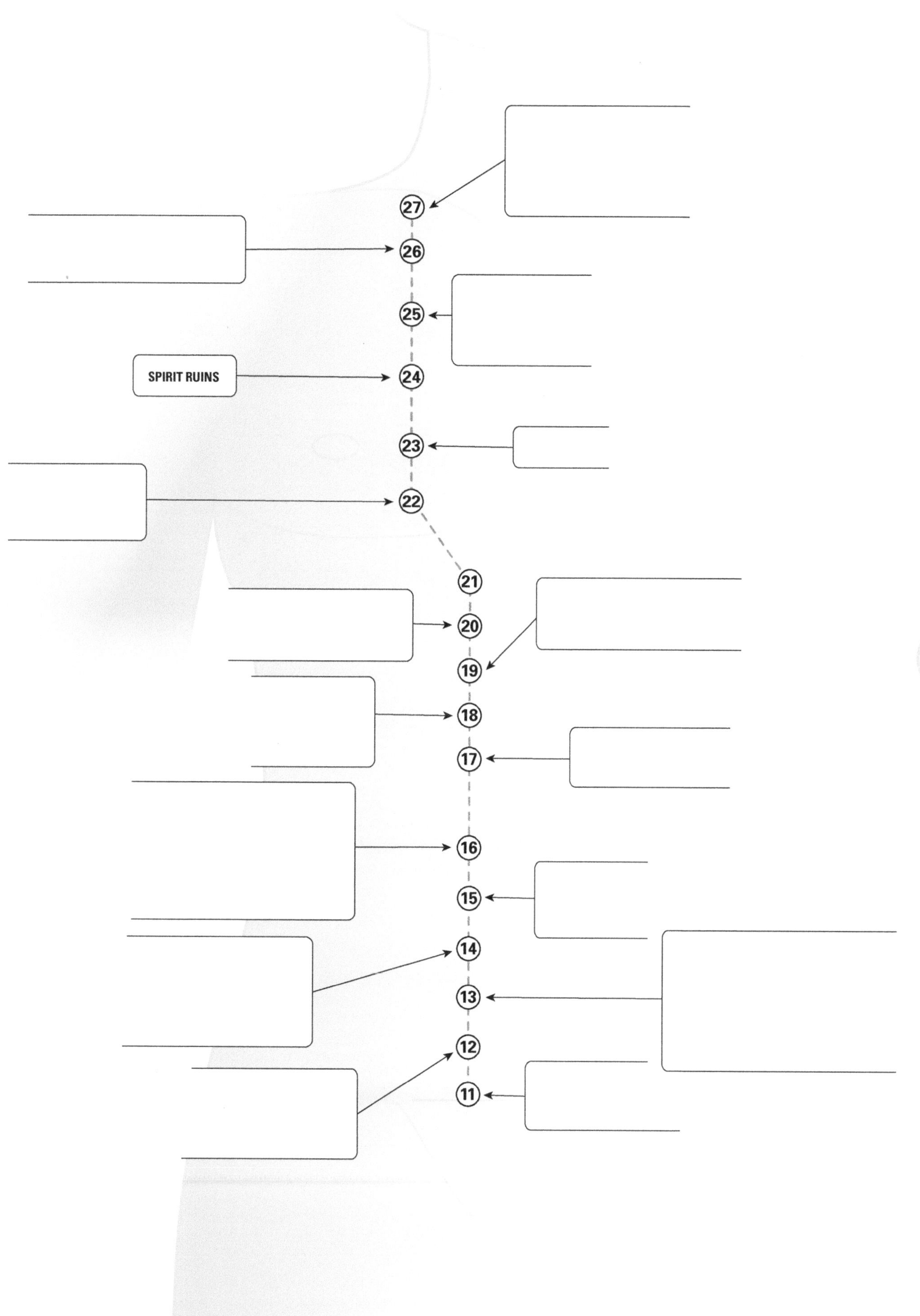
27
26
25
SPIRIT RUINS
24
23
22
21
20
19
18
17
16
15
14
13
12
11
KD
KIDNEY

1
2
3
4
5
6
7
8
9

PC

PERICARDIUM $\mathcal{FX}s$

LATERAL VIEW

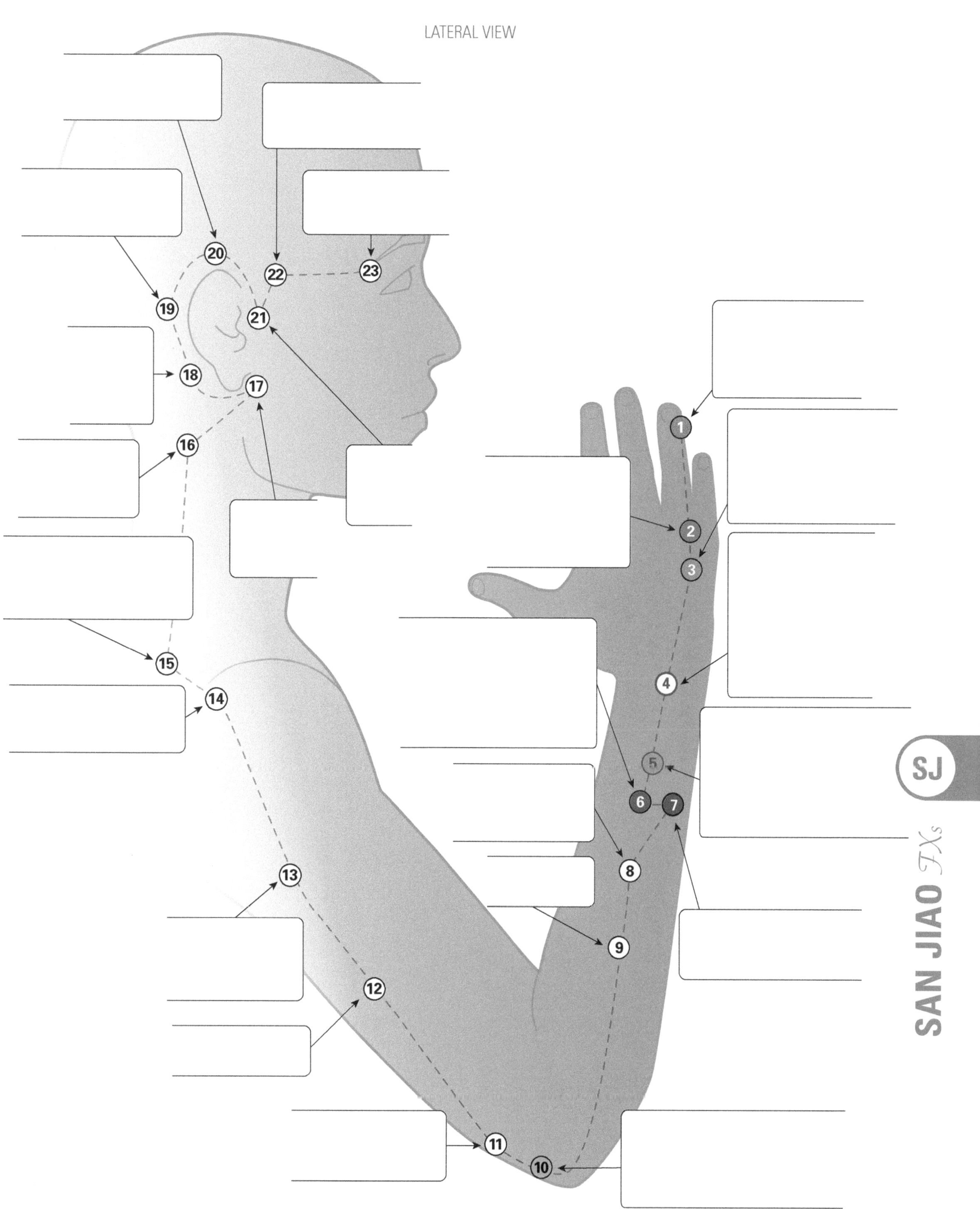

SJ

SAN JIAO FXs

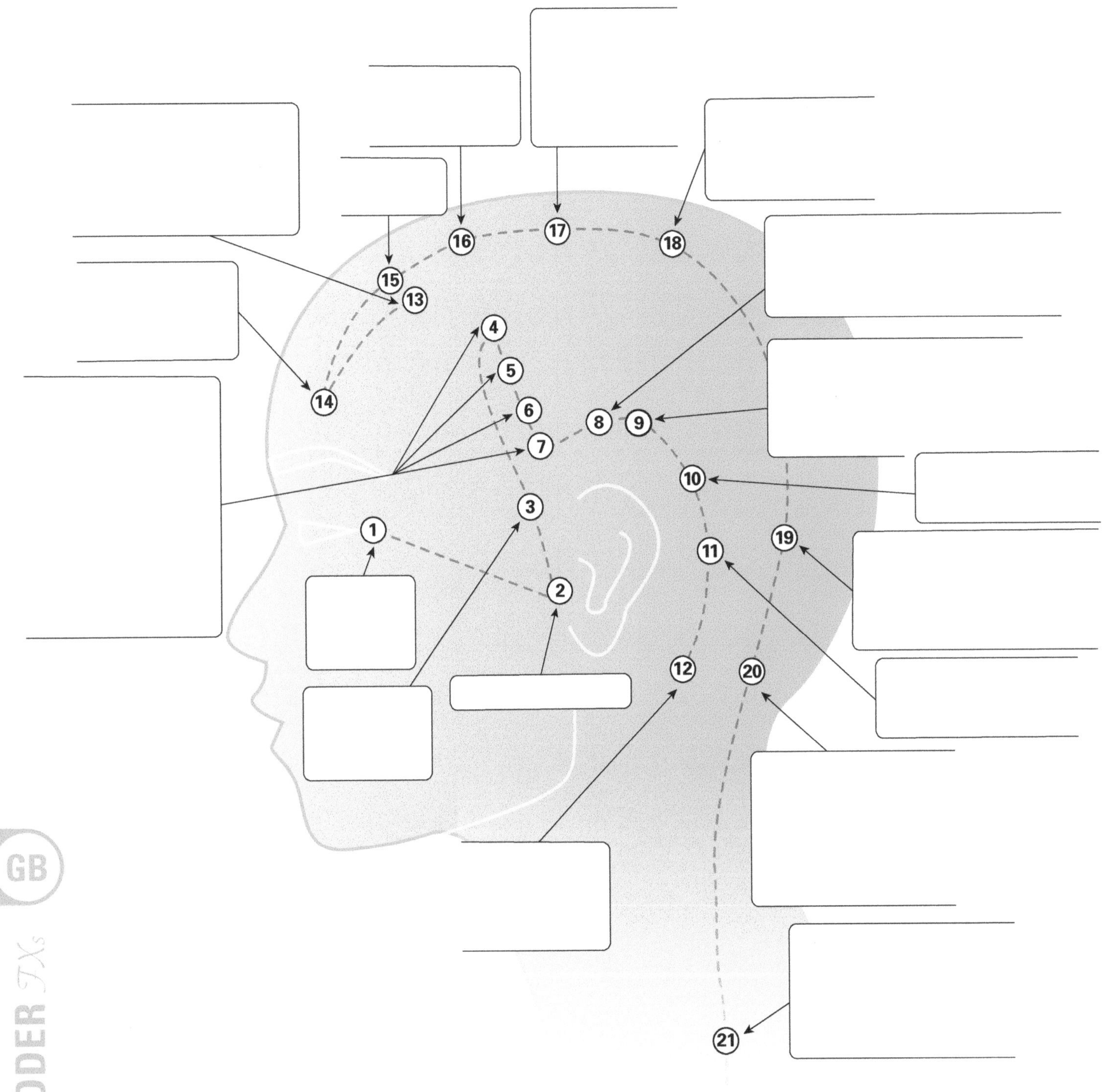
1
2
3
4
5
6
7
8
9
10
11
12
13
14
15
16
17
18
19
20
21

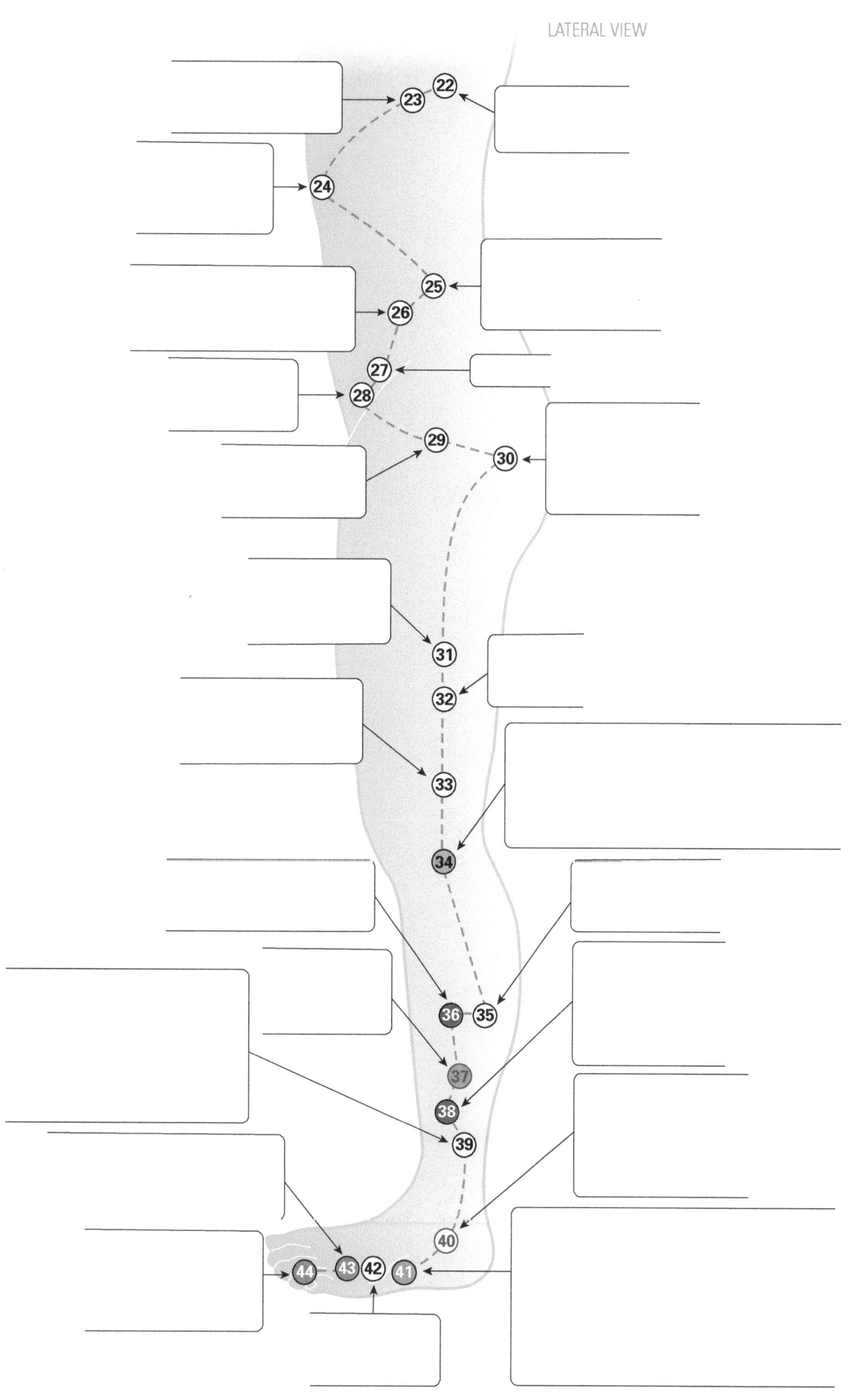
LATERAL VIEW
22
23
24
25
26
27
28
29
30
31
32
33
34
35
36
37
38
39
40
41
42
43
44

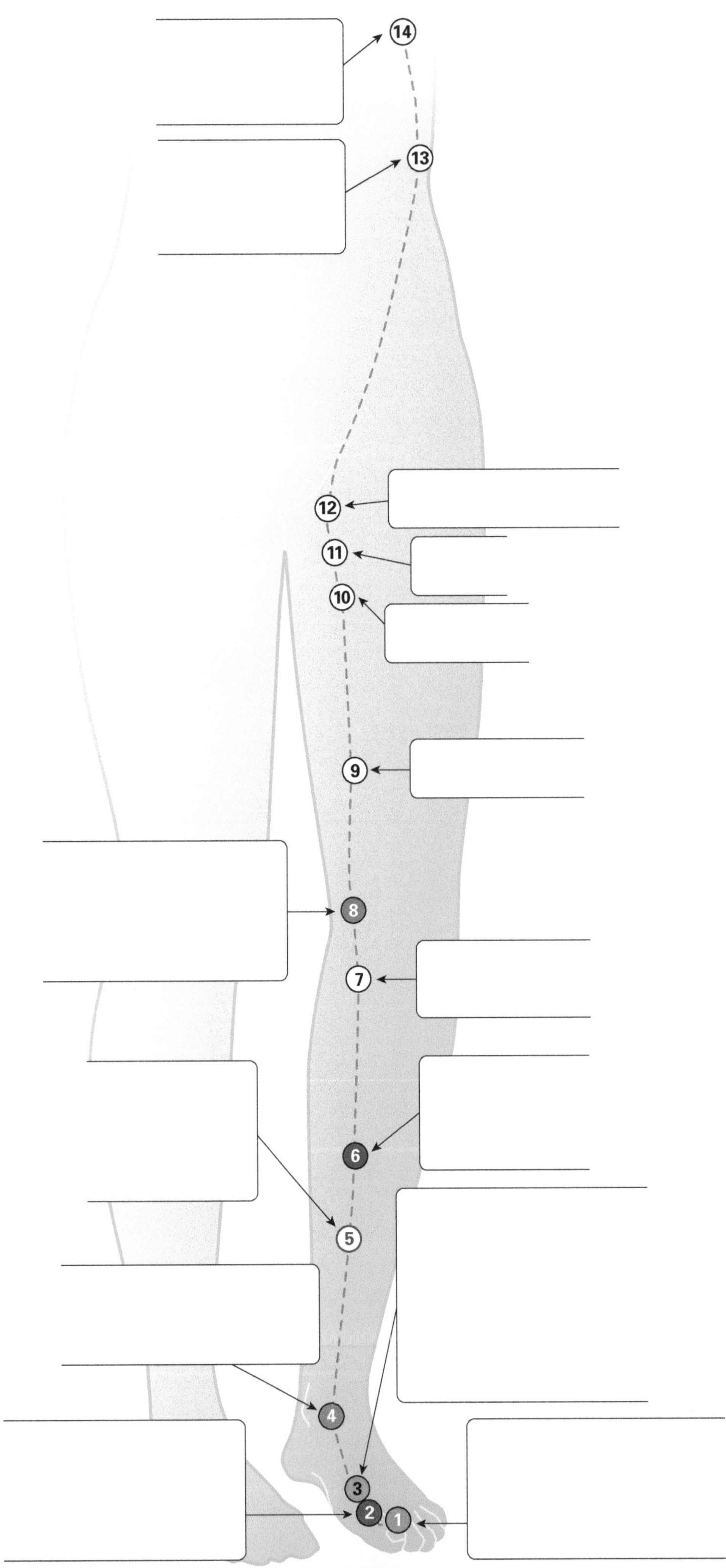

LV

LIVER $\mathcal{F}X_s$

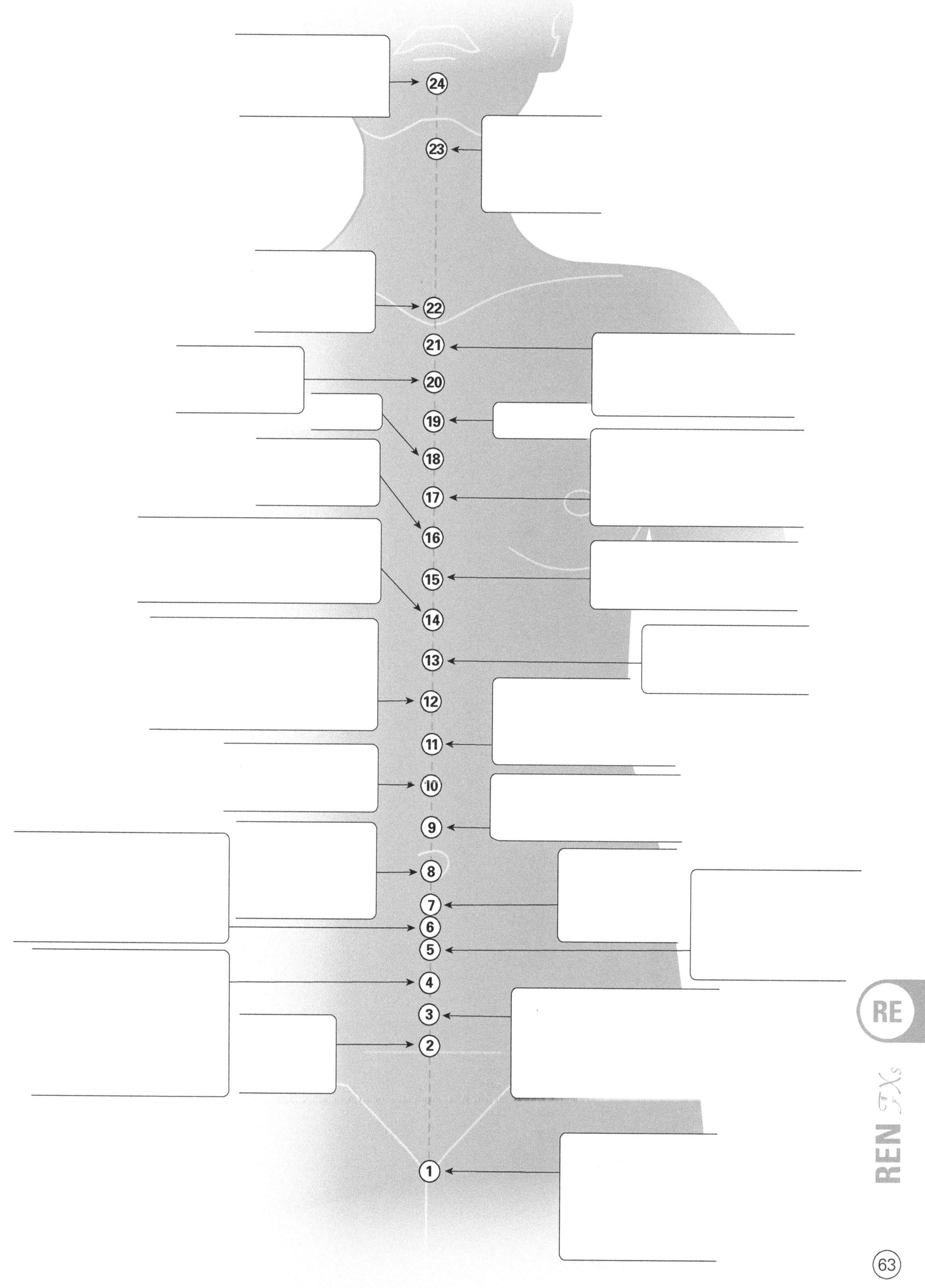
24
23
22
21
20
19
18
17
16
15
14
13
12
11
10
9
8
7
6
5
4
3
2
1

POSTERIOR VIEW

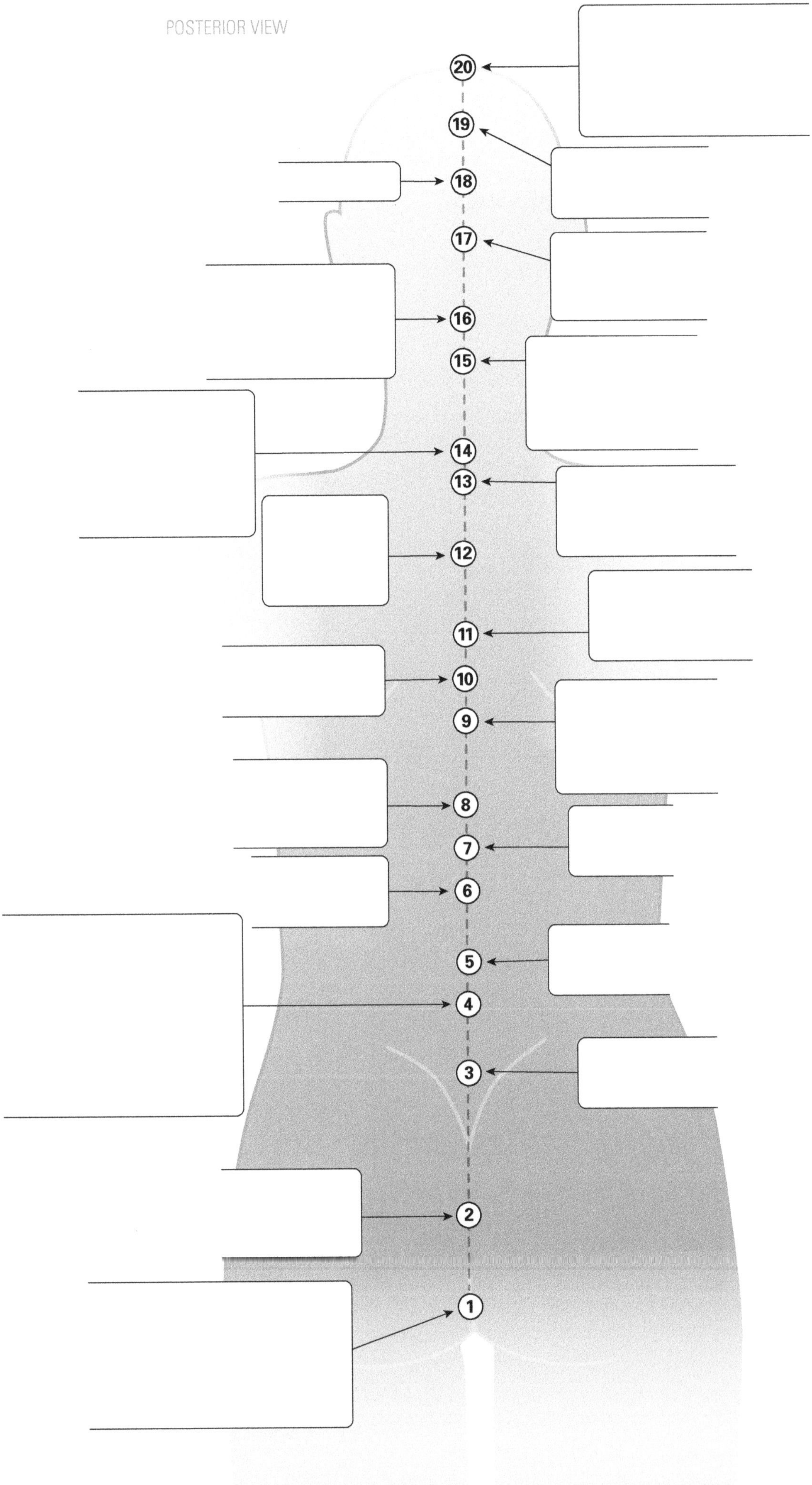

20

19

18

17

16

15

14

13

12

11

10

9

8

7

6

5

4

3

2

1

DU

DU $\mathcal{FX}_s$

ANTERIOR VIEW

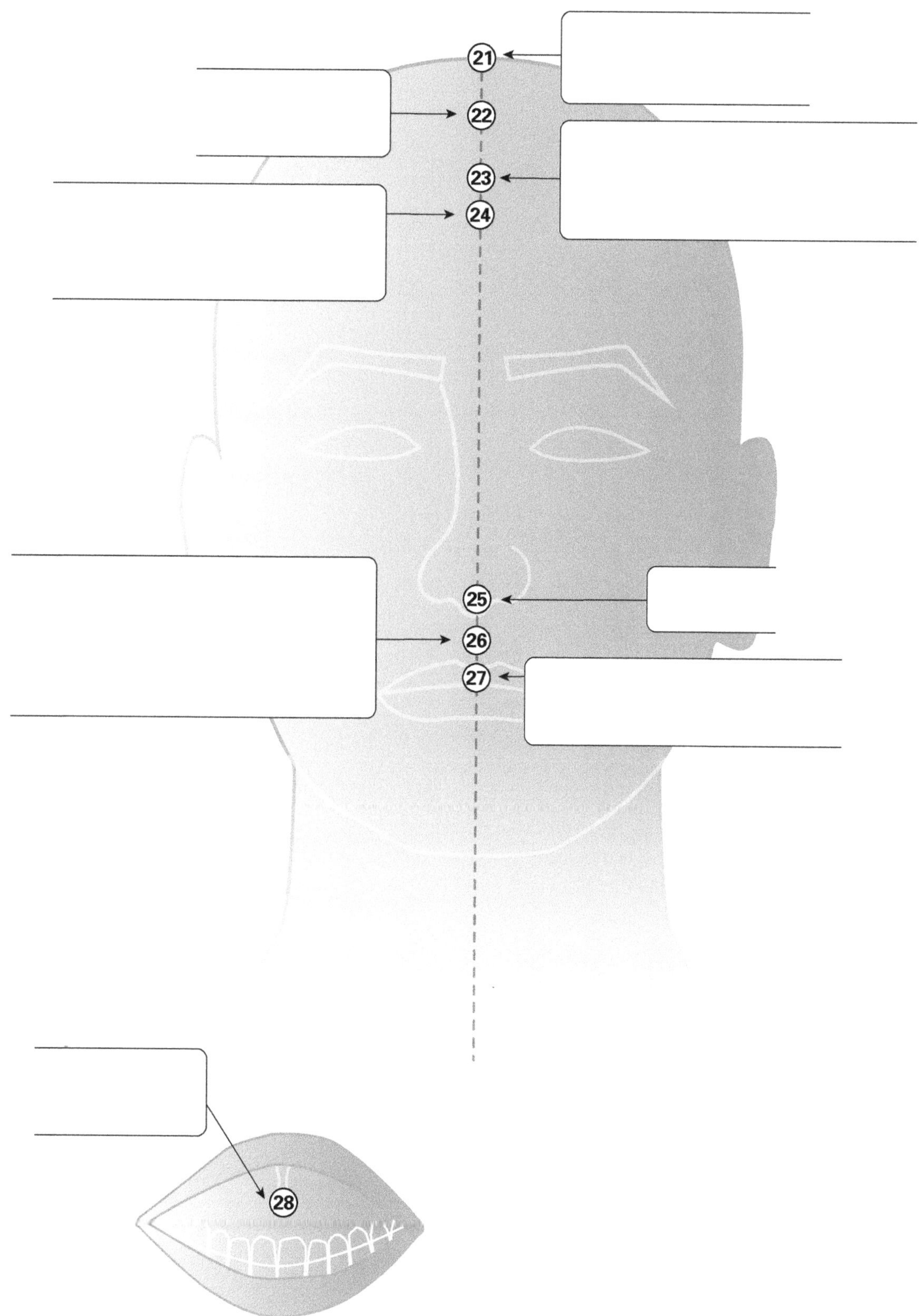

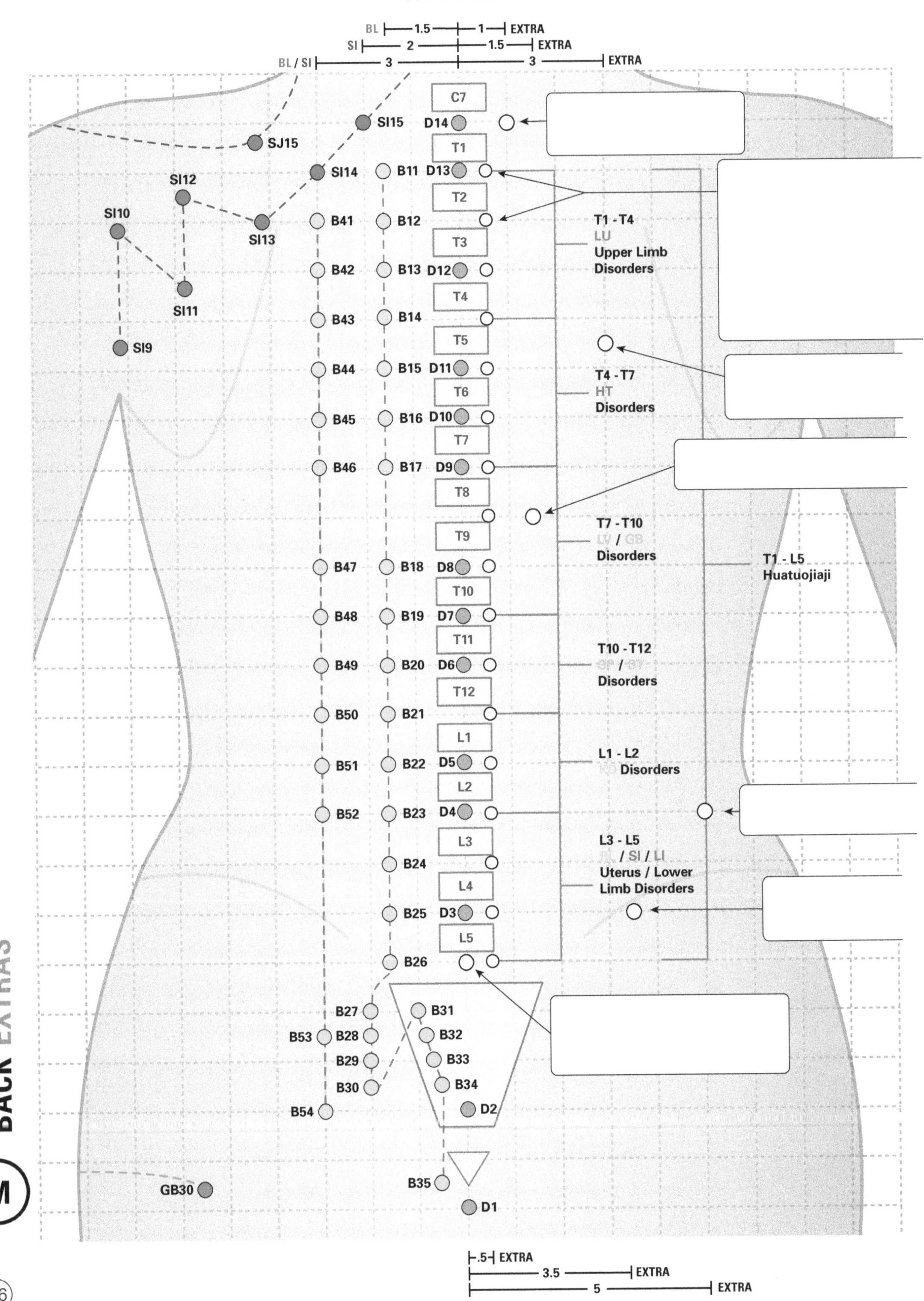

BACK EXTRAS

M

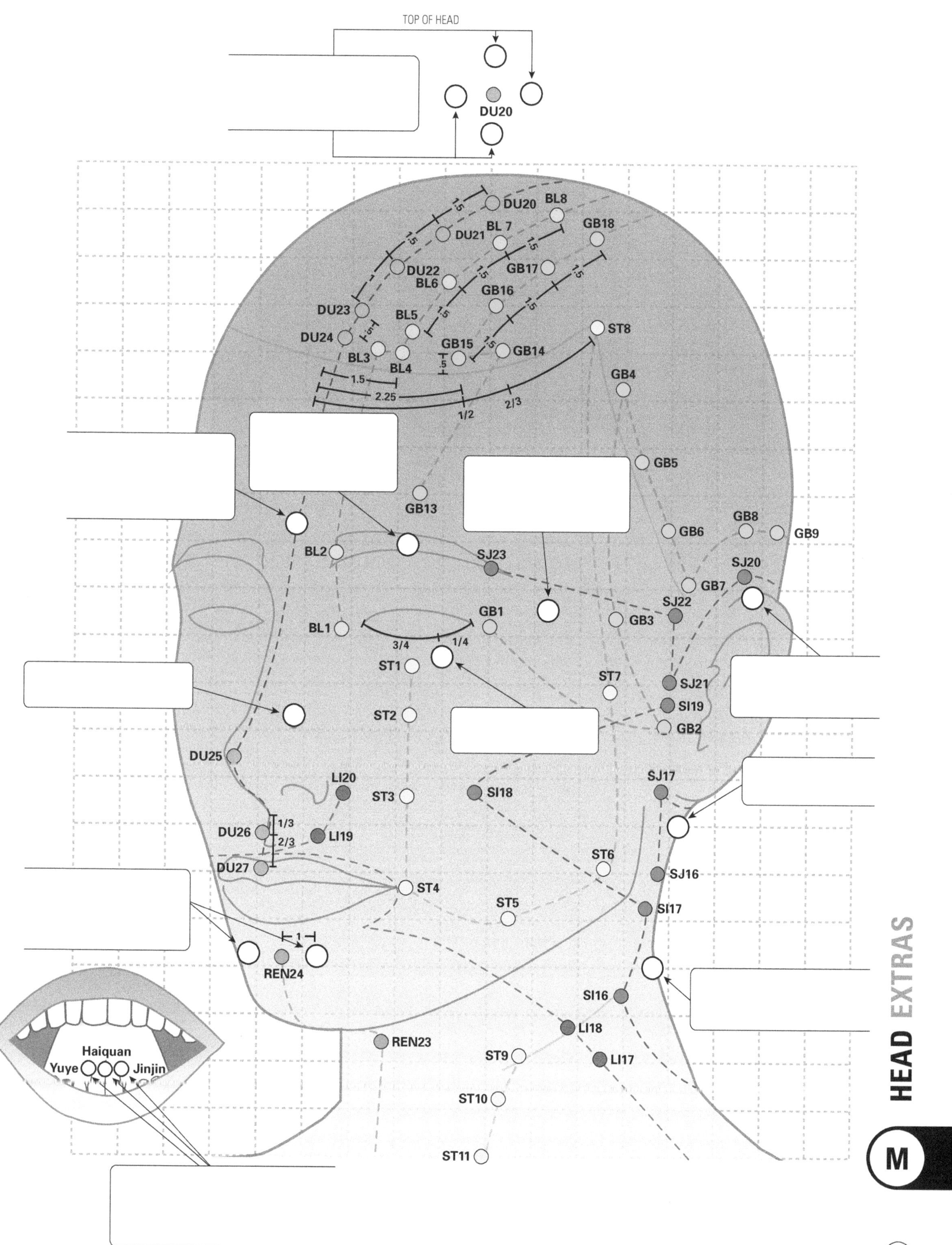
TOP OF HEAD
DU20
DU20
BL8
BL 7
GB18
DU21
DU22
BL6
GB17
GB16
DU23
BL5
DU24
BL3
BL4
GB15
GB14
ST8
GB4
1.5
2.25
1/2
2/3
GB5
GB13
GB8
GB6
GB9
BL2
SJ23
SJ20
GB7
SJ22
BL1
GB1
GB3
3/4
1/4
ST1
ST7
SJ21
SI19
ST2
GB2
DU25
LI20
SJ17
ST3
SI18
1/3
DU26
LI19
2/3
DU27
ST6
SJ16
ST4
ST5
SI17
1
REN24
SI16
LI18
REN23
Haiquan
Yuye
Jinjin
ST9
LI17
ST10
ST11

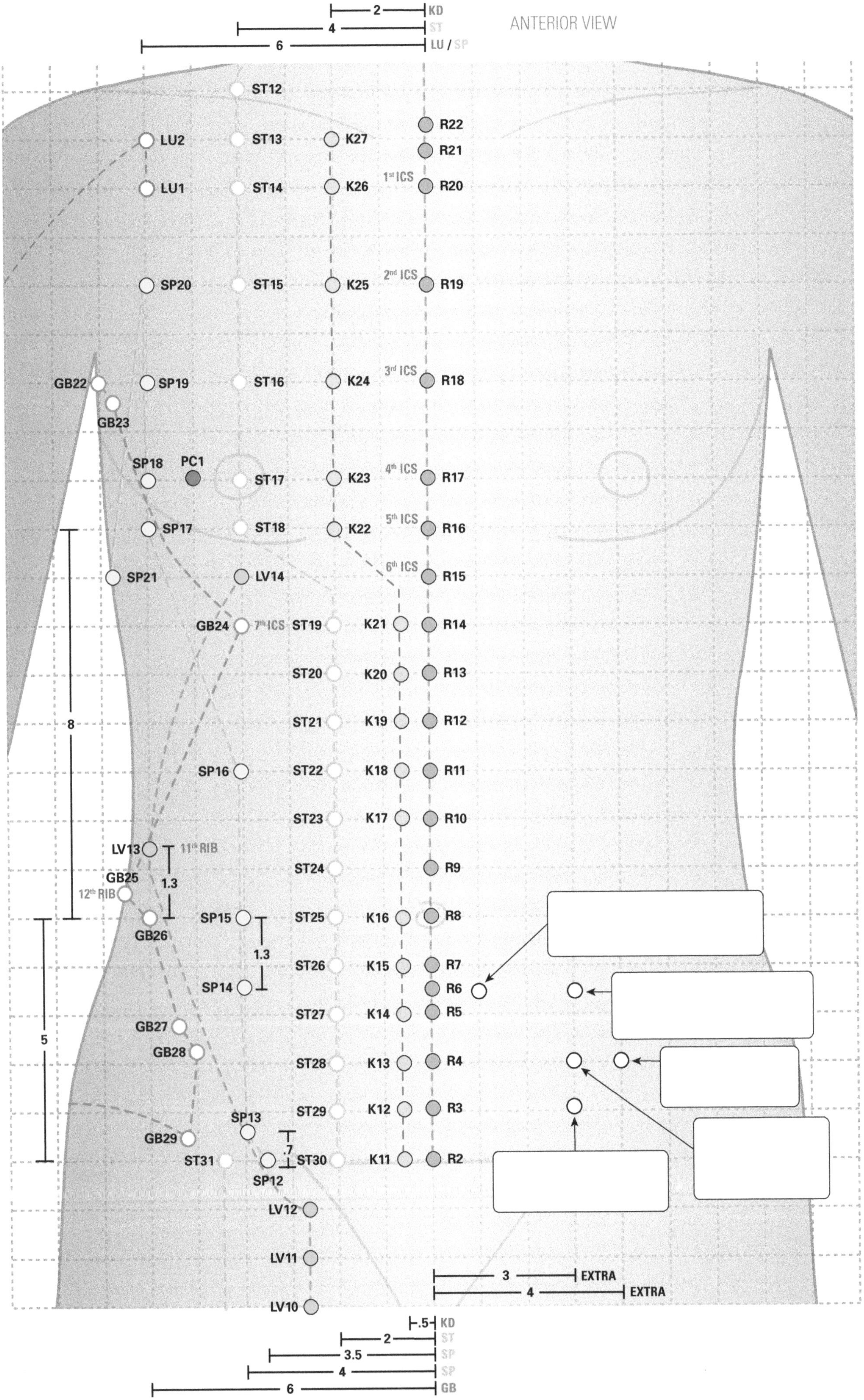

2 KD
4 ST
6 LU / SP

ST12
R22
LU2
ST13
K27
R21
1st ICS
LU1
ST14
K26
R20
SP20
ST15
K25
2nd ICS
R19
3rd ICS
GB22
SP19
ST16
K24
R18
GB23
SP18
PC1
4th ICS
ST17
K23
R17
5th ICS
SP17
ST18
K22
R16
6th ICS
SP21
LV14
R15
GB24
7th ICS
ST19
K21
R14
ST20
K20
R13
8
ST21
K19
R12
SP16
ST22
K18
R11
ST23
K17
R10
LV13
11th RIB
1.3
ST24
R9
GB25
12th RIB
SP15
ST25
K16
R8
GB26
1.3
ST26
K15
R7
SP14
R6
ST27
K14
R5
5
GB27
GB28
ST28
K13
R4
SP13
ST29
K12
R3
GB29
.7
ST31
ST30
K11
R2
SP12
LV12
LV11
3 EXTRA
4 EXTRA
LV10

.5 KD
2 ST
3.5 SP
4 SP
6 GB

TORSO EXTRAS

M

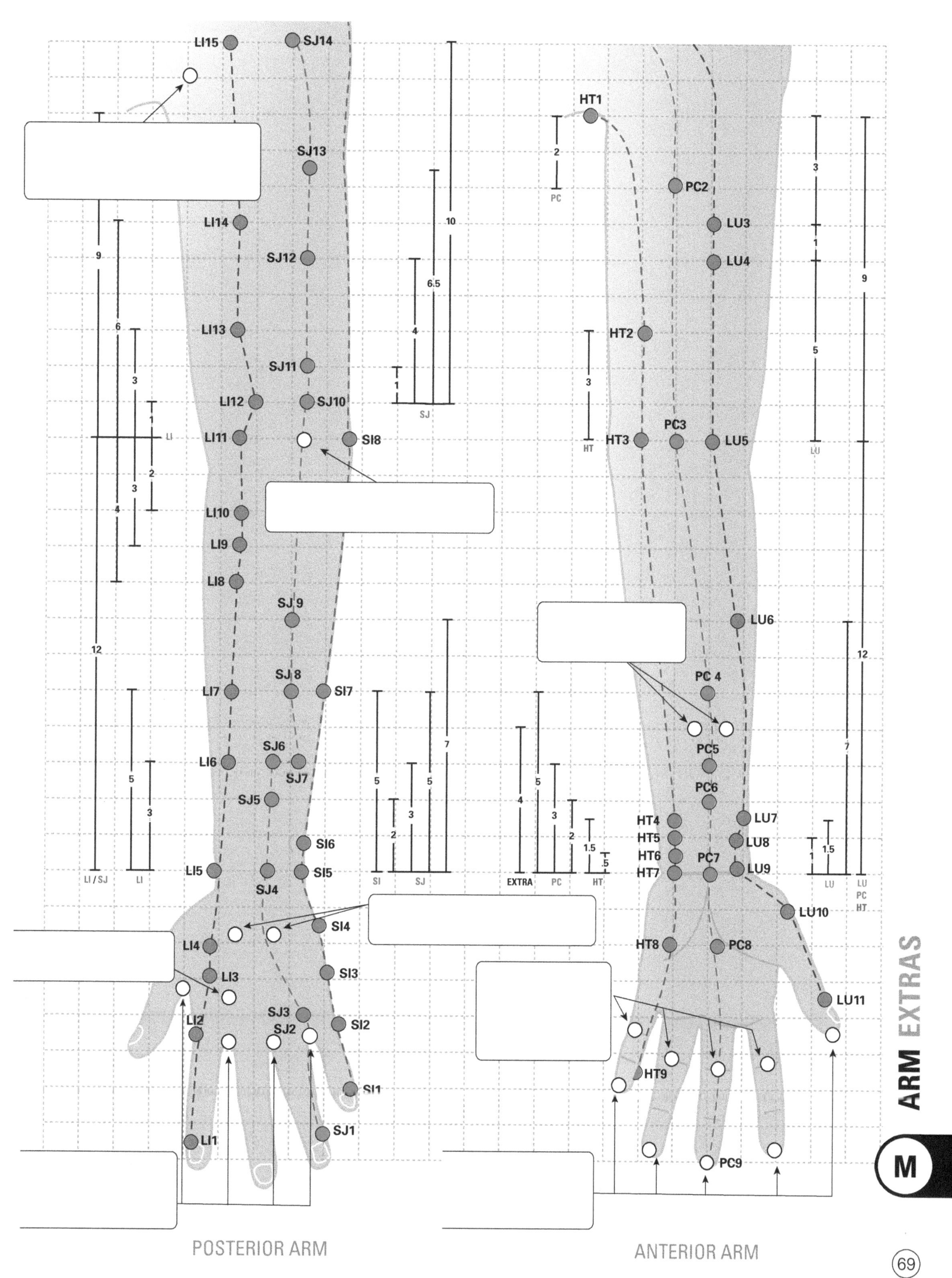

LI15
SJ14
SJ13
LI14
SJ12
LI13
SJ11
LI12
SJ10
LI11
SI8
LI10
LI9
LI8
SJ 9
SJ 8
LI7
SI7
SJ6
LI6
SJ7
SJ5
SI6
LI5
SJ4
SI5
SI4
LI4
LI3
SI3
SJ3
LI2
SJ2
SI2
SI1
SJ1
LI1
HT1
PC2
LU3
LU4
HT2
PC3
HT3
LU5
LU6
PC 4
PC5
PC6
HT4
HT5
HT6
HT7
PC7
LU7
LU8
LU9
LU10
HT8
PC8
LU11
HT9
PC9
POSTERIOR ARM
ANTERIOR ARM
ARM EXTRAS
M

LEG EXTRAS

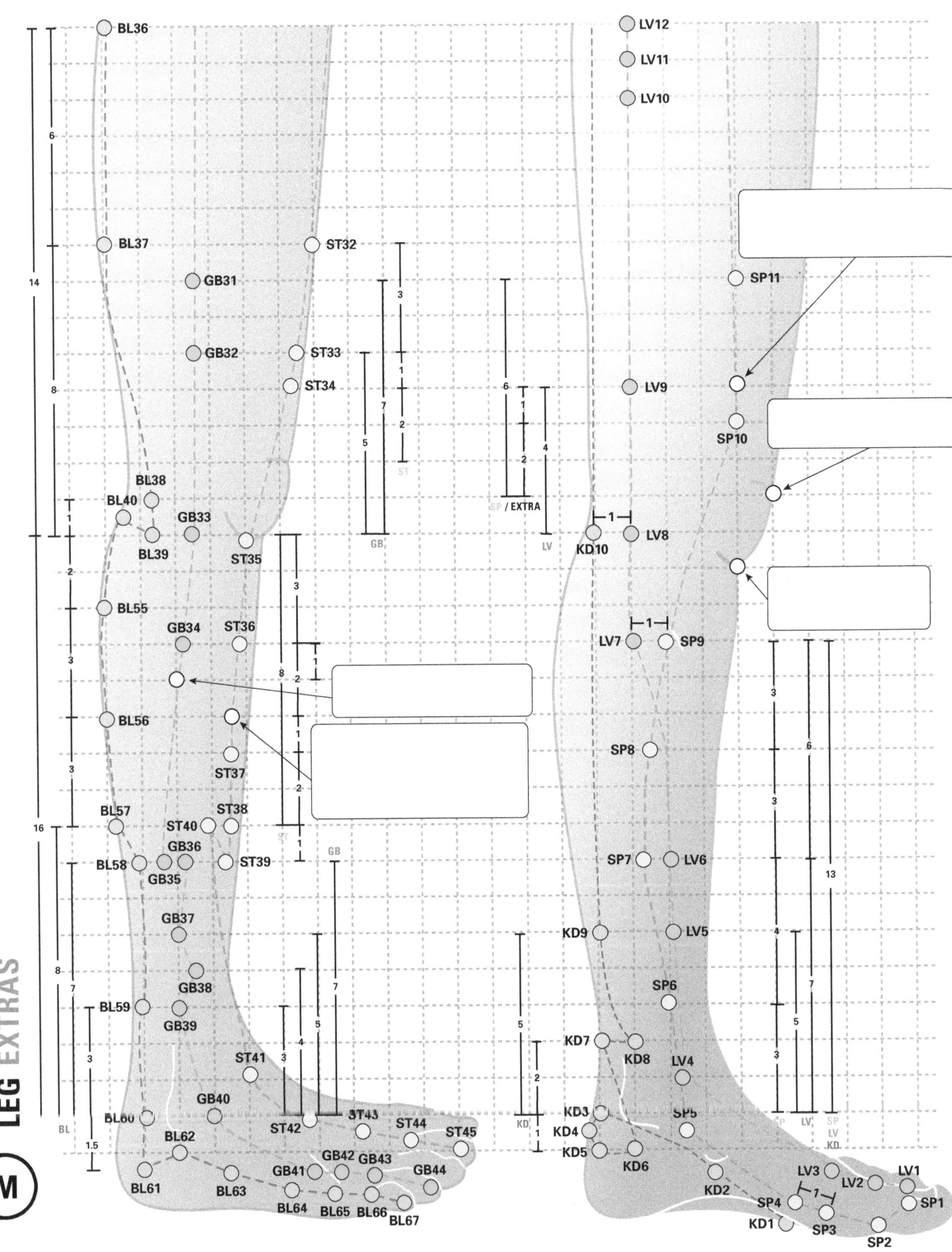

BL36
BL37
ST32
GB31
GB32
ST33
ST34
BL38
BL40
GB33
BL39
ST35
BL55
GB34
ST36
BL56
ST37
BL57
ST40
ST38
GB36
BL58
GB35
ST39
GB37
GB38
BL59
GB39
ST41
GB40
BL60
ST42
ST43
ST44
ST45
BL62
GB42
GB43
GB44
GB41
BL61
BL63
BL64
BL65
BL66
BL67
LV12
LV11
LV10
SP11
LV9
SP10
KD10
LV8
LV7
SP9
SP8
SP7
LV6
KD9
LV5
SP6
KD7
KD8
LV4
KD3
SP5
KD4
KD5
KD6
KD2
LV3
LV2
LV1
SP4
SP1
KD1
SP3
SP2
SP / EXTRA
LATERAL POSTERIOR
MEDIAL ANTERIOR